Recent Results in Cancer Research 105

Founding Editor
P. Rentchnick, Geneva

Managing Editors
Ch. Herfarth, Heidelberg · H. J. Senn, St. Gallen

Associate Editors
M. Baum, London · V. Diehl, Köln
C. von Essen, Villigen · E. Grundmann, Münster
W. Hitzig, Zürich · M. F. Rajewsky, Essen

Recent Results in Cancer Research

Breast Cancer

Present Perspective of Early Diagnosis

Edited by S. Brünner and B. Langfeldt

With 59 Figures and 43 Tables

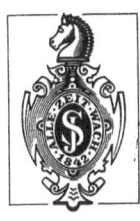

Springer-Verlag
Berlin Heidelberg New York
London Paris Tokyo

Assoc. Professor Sam Brünner, MD, PhD
Department of Diagnostic Radiology
Gentofte Hospital, University of Copenhagen
2900 Hellerup/Copenhagen, Denmark

Assoc. Professor Bent Langfeldt, MD, EDR
Department of Diagnostic Radiology
The County Hospital, University of Aarhus
8000 Aarhus, C., Denmark

ISBN-13:978-3-642-82966-6   e-ISBN-13:978-3-642-82964-2
DOI: 10.1007/978-3-642-82964-2

Library of Congress Cataloging-in-Publication Data.
Breast cancer. (Recent results in cancer research; 105) Based on the Third International
Copenhagen Symposium on Detection of Breast Cancer held in 1985. Includes biblio-
graphies and index. 1. Breast-Cancer-Diagnosis-Congresses. I. Brünner, Sam, 1920-   .
II. Langfeldt, B. (Bent), 1923-   . III. International Copenhagen Symposium on Detection
of Breast Cancer (3rd: 1985) IV. Series. [DNLM: 1. Breast Neoplasms-diagnosis-congresses.
W1 RE106P v. 105/WP 870 B8237 1985] RC261.R35 vol.105 616.99'4s 86-31459
[RC280.B8] [616.99'449075]

© Springer-Verlag Berlin Heidelberg 1987
Softcover reprint of the hardcover 1st edition   1987

2125/3140-543210

Preface

The Third International Copenhagen Symposium on Detection of Breast Cancer afforded a further opportunity for scientists from all over the world to come together and present important papers concerning breast cancer and early diagnostic procedures. The Symposium was an opportunity to learn from extensive screening procedures carried out at outstanding centers in the United States, Sweden, the Netherlands, and England. Furthermore, the Symposium dealt with new modalities such as ultrasonography, magnification techniques, and magnetic resonance; and very important contributions concerning self-examination, fine needle aspiration biopsy, and radiation risks were presented. A whole section was also dedicated to the highly important cooperation between radiologist, surgeon, and pathologist. It is our sincere hope that a study of the different aspects of breast cancer presented in this volume will encourage the reader to join in the struggle against this dreadful disease.

December 1986   S. Brünner
                                                             B. Langfeldt

Contents

VIII   Contents

List of Contributors*

Andersson, I. 62[1]

Andersen, J.A. 97, 124

Beckmann, J. 73

Beckmann, M. 73

Blichert-Toft, M. 97

Brünner, S. 73

Christensen, L. 124

Dyreborg, U. 124

Feig, S.A. 15, 25, 78, 85, 89, 111

Frasca, P. 25

Galkin, B.M. 15, 25, 89, 111

Gästrin, G. 106

Haus, A.G. 37

Jakobsen, S. 73

Muir, H.D. 15, 25, 89, 111

Nielsen, B. 1

Nielsen, M. 124

Patchefsky, A.S. 89

Price, J.L. 67

Sickles, E.A. 19, 31, 52

Sigfússon, B.F. 62

Soriano, R.Z. 25

Svane, G. 95

Tabár, L. 58

Thomas, B.A. 67

Watt-Boolsen, S. 97

West Andersen, K. 97

---

* The address of the principal author is given on the first page of each contribution.

[1] Page on which contribution begins.

Image Quality in Mammography:
Physical and Technical Limitations

B. Nielsen

Department of Radiation Physics, University of Linköping, 58185 Linköping, Sweden

Introduction

Special imaging problems arise in mammography since the conditions are quite different from those in other fields of radiology. The differences in attenuation of the various soft tissue structures in the female breast are small, and it is necessary to use X-rays with low photon energy in order to get a sufficiently high contrast in the mammographic film. Jennings and Fewell (1979) examined the relative exposure necessary to achieve a constant signal-to-noise ratio for various photon energies. They found a minimum at approximately 20 keV, when glandular tissue in the breast was imaged. Moreover, small details such as microcalcifications may have diameters no larger than 0.1 mm and can only be imaged using a system with high spatial resolution. Although microcalcifications have high attenuation, their small dimensions along the direction of the X-ray beam reduce their attenuation so that it is necessary to use a system giving high contrast.

Special attention has been paid to the absorbed dose and the risk of carcinogenesis in the breast from mammography (Feig 1983; Hammerstein et al. 1979; Lester 1977; Muntz 1979; NCRP 1980; Stanton et al. 1984; ICRP 1983). This has made the imaging task even more complicated. In recent years, screening asymptomatic women with mammography – sometimes with a limited number of views per breast – has further emphasized the need for high-quality low-dose mammography.

Film-screen mammography is a well-established technique in which great interest has been shown in the past (Friedrich and Weskamp 1976; Friedrich 1978; Gould and Genant 1981; Muntz 1979b; Jennings et al. 1981; DeSmet et al. 1982; Haus 1984). The mammographic technique has been under continuous development, and extensive studies of the choice of film screen combination, spatial resolution, and contrast exist.

For a long time the effect of scattered radiation was neglected in mammography, since it was believed that the amount of scatter was very small. However, many authors (Lammers and Kuhn 1979; Muntz 1979a; King et al. 1979; Yester et al. 1981) have pointed out that scatter reduction is also important in mammography.

On the Choice of Spectral Distribution, Filtration, and Anode Material

Today the most common anode material in X-ray tubes used in mammography is molybdenum in combination with a thin molybdenum filter. This gives the necessary low-energy spectrum needed. An example of a primary mammographic spectrum at 30 kV_p with a molybdenum anode can be seen in Fig. 1. The primary data were taken from Birch et al. (1979).

Recent Results in Cancer Research. Vol 105
© Springer-Verlag Berlin · Heidelberg 1987

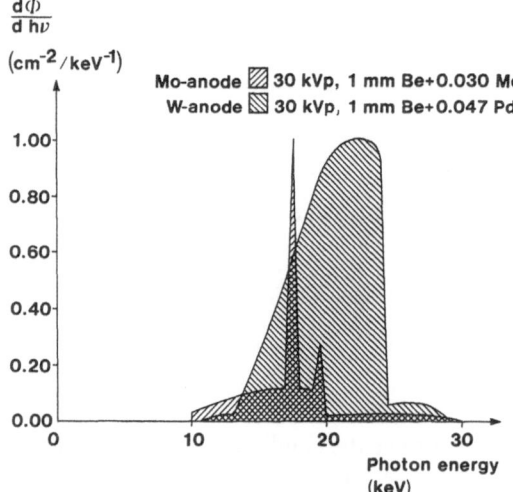

$$\frac{d\phi}{d\,h\nu}$$

(cm^{-2}/keV^{-1})

Mo-anode ▨ 30 kVp, 1 mm Be+0.030 Mo
W-anode ▨ 30 kVp, 1 mm Be+0.047 Pd

Fig. 1. Primary mammographic spectra at 30 kV$_p$ accelerating tube potential for a molybdenum tube with a 0.030-mm molybdenum filter and a tungsten tube with a 0.047-mm palladium filter

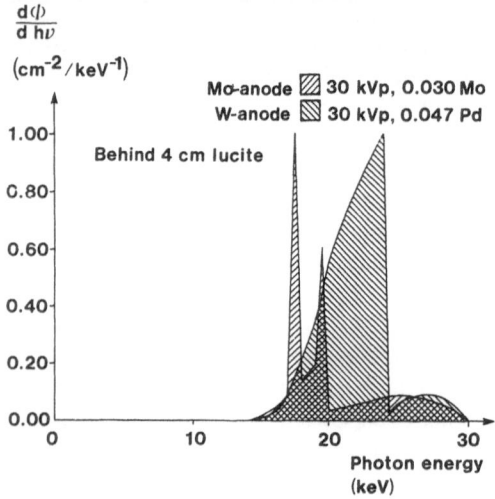

$$\frac{d\phi}{d\,h\nu}$$

(cm^{-2}/keV^{-1})

Mo-anode ▨ 30 kVp, 0.030 Mo
W-anode ▨ 30 kVp, 0.047 Pd

Behind 4 cm lucite

Fig. 2. Primary photon spectra at 30 kV$_p$ tube potential attenuated by 4 cm of lucite: molybdenum anode with 0.030 mm molybdenum, tungsten anode with 0.047 mm palladium

Recently, it has been suggested that X-ray tubes with tungsten anodes used with palladium filters would give images comparable to those of molybdenum tubes (Beaman and Lillicrap 1982; Beaman et al. 1983; McDonagh et al. 1984). An example of a primary mammographic spectrum at 30 kV$_p$ with a tungsten anode is also shown in Fig. 1, from which it can be seen that the molybdenum tube gives a spectrum containing more low-energy photons than the tungsten tube. For thin objects, the molybdenum anode tube must therefore be superior from the point of view of primary contrast. This is in agreement with the findings of Beaman et al. (1983). In Fig. 2 the same primary photon spectra as in Fig. 1 are shown after being attenuated in 4 cm of lucite.

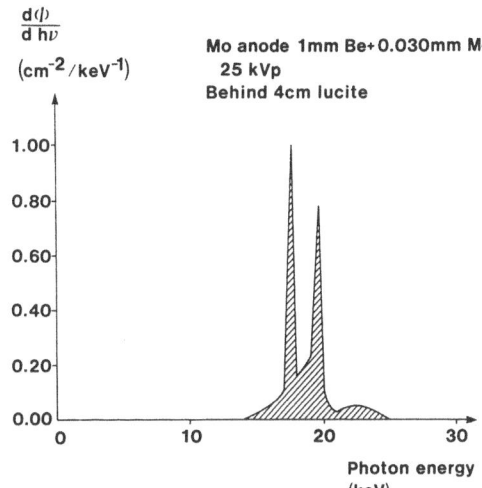

$$\frac{d\phi}{d\,h\nu}$$

(cm^{-2}/keV^{-1})

Mo anode 1mm Be+0.030mm Mo
25 kVp
Behind 4cm lucite

1.00
0.80
0.60
0.40
0.20
0.00

0   10   20   30

Photon energy
(keV)

Fig. 3. Molybdenum spectra at 25 kV$_p$ after attenuation in 4 cm lucite

From Figs. 1 and 2, it can be seen that placing an object in the beam heavily attenuates the molybdenum-characteristic radiation peaks and increases the relative importance of the bremsstrahlung spectra, thus decreasing image contrast. This is the reason for the choice of the low accelerating potential used with Mo anode tubes. In Fig. 3, the spectrum for a Mo tube at 25 kV$_p$ accelerating potential attenuated by 4 cm lucite is shown.

A comparison of the Mo spectra of Figs. 2 and 3 clearly shows the reduced bremsstrahlung contribution at 25 kV$_p$.

Data from Jennings and Fewell (1979) show that for a 5-cm-thick phantom of lucite, the mean energy determined from the measured photon fluence spectra of the molybdenum anode tube at 30 kV$_p$ is lower that for the tungsten tube, the values being 21.1 and 22.4 keV respectively. For even thicker phantoms the effective energy is similar for Mo tubes and W tubes.

McDonagh et al. (1984) showed that for a breast thickness of 3–4 cm the Mo tube was the optimal, while for both thinner and thicker breasts the optimum choice was the W tube together with a K-edge filter of rhodium or niobium.

The effect of voltage waveform on output and penetration has been studied by O'Foghludha and Johnson (1981). They found that the difference in output for full wave rectification (100% ripple) and constant potential (no ripple) was a factor of two in favor of the constant potential technique with both Mo and W tubes.

The penetration (and hence indirectly the contrast) is only slightly affected by the waveform for a Mo tube, while it has a strong influence for the W tube, with higher penetration at the constant potential. The gain in practice of the waveform effect is believed to be limited because the ripple on a 6-pulse unit (the most common units today) is theoretically only 13%.

Image Quality Limitations in the Standard Mammographic Technique

Spatial Resolution

In the standard mammographic technique (Fig. 4), the breast is pressed against the cassette and the distance between the object and the film is small. For a typical distance be-

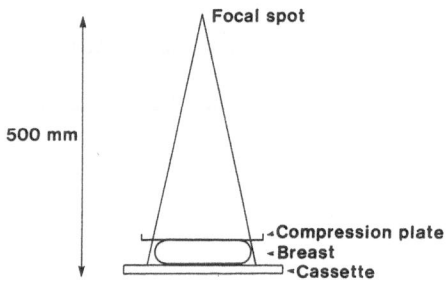

Magnification: 1.03-1.08

Fig. 4. Geometrical principles of the standard mammographic technique

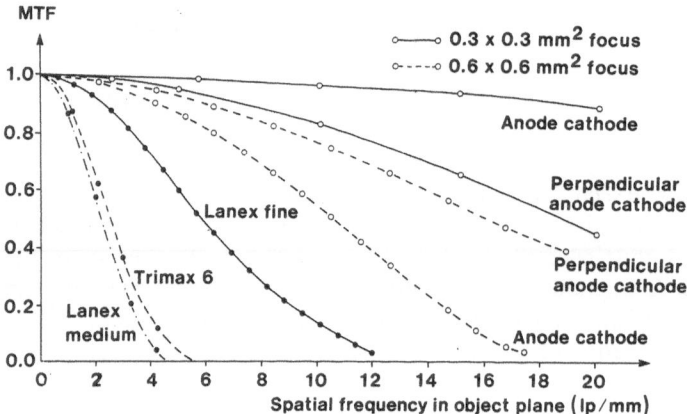

Fig. 5. The modulation transfer function for two focal spots and three fluorescent screens. For the focal spots, the MTFs are shown in orthogonal directions

tween the focal spot and the film of 500 mm, the magnification is between 1.03 and 1.08, being, e. g., 1.05 for a test object placed 25 mm above the cassette.

We have used the modulation transfer function, MTF (Rossmann 1964), for the imaging components as a tool in optimizing spatial resolution. MTFs were calculated as Fourier transforms of the line spread function (Rossmann 1964). The line spread function was obtained by microdensitometric scanning of a pinhole image recorded on film. A correction for the pinhole MTF was applied. For screen-film systems, the line spread function was linearized by the measured characteristic curves of the films.

In Fig. 5, the modulation transfer functions for a 0.3×0.3 mm^2 and a 0.6×0.6 mm^2 focal spot at $1.05 \times$ magnification are shown together with the MTFs for some common fluorescent screens used as single back screens. It can be seen that even for the 0.6×0.6 mm^2 focal spot, the fluorescent screen is the factor limiting the spatial resolution obtainable.

Note: The MTF curves in Fig. 5 show that the 0.3×0.3 mm^2 focal spot has its highest spatial resolution in the direction parallel to the anode-cathode direction, while the 0.6×0.6 mm^2 focal spot gives its highest spatial resolution in the direction perpendicular to the anode-cathode. This is due to a difference in the construction of the two particular mammographic X-ray tubes tested.

In Fig. 6, the total MTFs for the systems are calculated. It can be seen that there is an improvement in MTF if the 0.3×0.3 mm^2 focal spot is used with the standard technique.

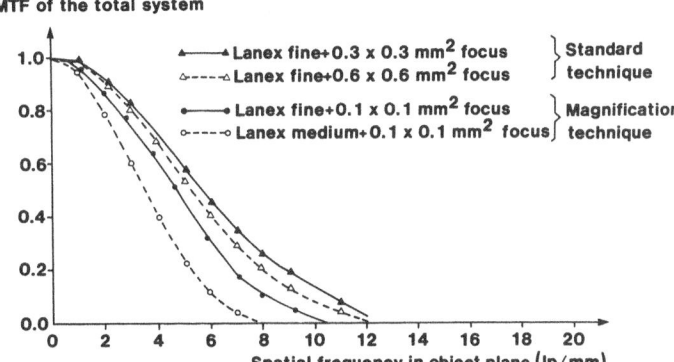

Fig. 6. Total MTFs for the mammographic standard and magnification techniques. In the calculations, the focal spot direction with the poorer spatial resolution has been used

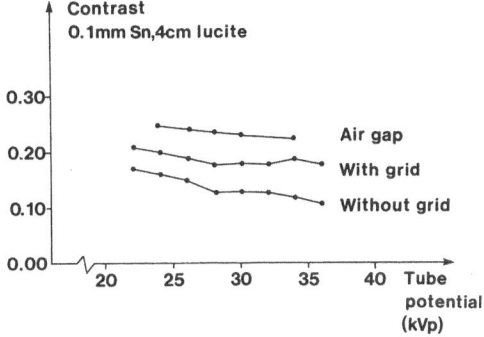

Fig. 7. The contrast for a 100-μm tin *(Sn)* foil embedded in a 4-cm lucite phantom as a function of tube potential, with a moving grid and without grid, and with the magnification technique (25-cm *air gap*). Mo tube with 0.030-mm Mo filter. Grid data: ratio 5, 30 lines/cm

Thus, in the standard mammographic technique, the spatial resolution can be said to be limited by the spatial resolution of the screen.

The MTF curves in Figs. 5 and 6 are in good agreement with the work of Bassett et al. (1981) and Arnold et al. (1979).

Contrast

The contrast obtained using the standard mammographic technique is determined by the tube potential, scattered radiation, and film gradient. The influence of the tube potential can be seen in Fig. 7. The precision of the contrast was estimated to be ±4%.

As can be seen from Fig. 7, increasing the tube potential decreases the contrast. An increase of the tube potential from 25 to 30 kV$_p$ decreases the contrast by approximately 10% whether or not a grid is used. The lowest tube potential used today is 25 kV$_p$. Still lower tube potentials would give unacceptably long exposure times.

From Fig. 7, it can also be seen that there is a great improvement in contrast when an anti-scatter grid is used as compared with the no-grid case. Even higher contrast can be obtained using an air gap, which also shows the same variation with tube potential as a grid.

Image Quality Limitations in Mammographic Magnification Technique

Spatial Resolution

When the magnification technique is used in mammography, the breast is normally moved closer to the X-ray tube, while keeping the distance between focus and film at approximately 500 mm. This is schematically shown in Fig. 8.

As in all magnification techniques, the focal spot size is the most critical parameter in determining the spatial resolution.

In Fig. 9, the MTF for a focal spot intended for the magnification technique with a nominal size 0.1 × 0.1 mm² is shown. Only the poorer direction is shown. For comparison, the MTFs for two common fluorescent screens are also shown.

It is apparent that, in combination with the Lanex fine screen, the focal spot size is the limiting factor at magnification 2.2.

The restricted loadability of microfocal spots makes the use of a faster screen-film combination desirable.

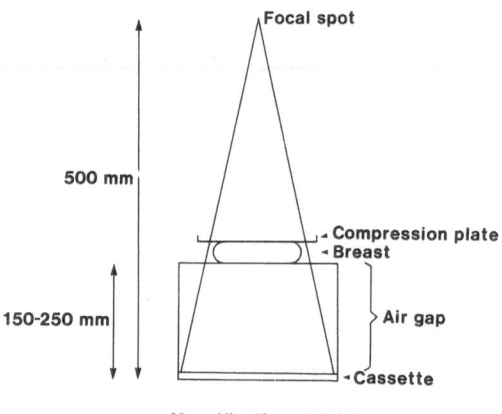

Fig. 8. Geometrical principles of the magnification technique

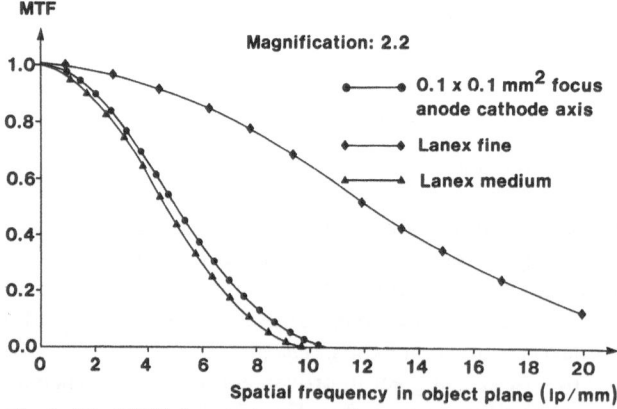

Fig. 9. The MTFs for two common fluorescent screens and for a focal spot used in the magnification technique

The Lanex medium screen is a reasonably good choice. In Fig. 6 the total MTFs for these two systems are shown, and it can be seen that the resulting improvement in spatial resolution obtained by using the Lanex fine screen in the magnification technique is substantial.

At present, Lanex fine screens cannot be used clinically with the magnification technique because of the long exposure times required.

Contrast

In the magnification technique the contrast is determined by tube potential and film gradient. The scattered radiation is effectively reduced by the air gap used. Quantitative data on this will be given in the next section. Due to tube loading restrictions, the minimum tube potential in current use with the magnification technique is 25 kV$_p$. The only way to improve image contrast is therefore to increase the film gradient. From Fig. 7, it can be seen that the contrast attained with the magnification technique is superior to that obtained by both no-grid and grid techniques.

Noise

Although noise in the mammographic image is not emphasized in this work, the noise is substantially reduced in magnified images (Doi and Imhof 1977).

The low photon energy used in mammography reduces quantum noise in comparison to standard radiography. However, we still consider that reducing noise with magnification is important particularly as regards the detection of microcalcifications.

Ratios of Imparted Energies Due to Scattered and Primary Radiation

Scattered radiation determines the contrast C of an image according to the relation (Morgan 1946; Wagner et al. 1980; Nielsen and Carlsson 1984):

$$C = D_2 - D_1 = \frac{C_p}{1 + \dfrac{\varepsilon_s}{\varepsilon_p}} \tag{1}$$

where D_1 and D_2 are respectively the optical densities of a film behind and beside a thin contrast detail. C and C_p are the contrasts with and without scattered radiation. ε_s and ε_p are the energies imparted to a small element of the fluorescent screen by scattered and primary radiation.

From Eq. 1, it can be seen that if the $\varepsilon_s/\varepsilon_p$ ratio amounts to 0.5, the contrast is reduced to 67% of the primary contrast value. An $\varepsilon_s/\varepsilon_p$ ratio of 0.5 is typical for mammography without scatter reduction. Scattered radiation is therefore an important factor in determining contrast even in mammography.

Scatter to primary ratios were measured with a lead beam stop in front of a lucite phantom. The optical densities beside and behind the lead beam stop were converted to energies imparted to the fluorescent screen using the film characteristic curve. The energy imparted from primary radiation was found by subtracting the scattered signal from the total (primary and scattered).

In Fig. 10, the scatter to primary ratio obtained at 25 kV$_p$ for different lucite thicknesses is shown, with and without grid, for a field size of 18×24 cm². The accuracy of the $\varepsilon_s/\varepsilon_p$ ratio without a grid was estimated to be $\pm 5\%$.

From Fig. 10, it can be seen that the $\varepsilon_s/\varepsilon_p$ ratio increases when the phantom thickness is increased. With approximately 5.5 cm lucite, the $\varepsilon_s/\varepsilon_p$ ratio is 1.0 without grid, i.e., the contrast is reduced to 50% of the primary contrast value. When a grid is employed, the $\varepsilon_s/\varepsilon_p$ ratio is more or less constant with increasing lucite thickness, with a tendency to increase at 5-6 cm lucite.

In Fig. 11 the scatter to primary ratio with constant phantom thickness is shown as a function of tube potential.

The scatter to primary ratios in Figs. 10 and 11 are in good agreement with the work of Dance and Day (1984). The difference between our results and those of Barnes and Brezovich (1978) can be explained by the fact that these authors used a smaller solid angle of acceptance for the detector and different detector materials.

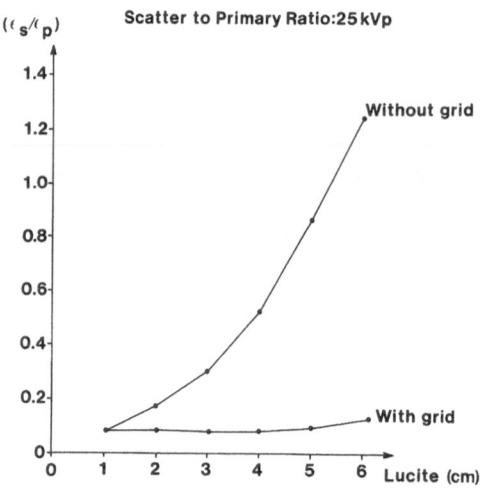

Fig. 10. Scatter to primary ratios obtained at 25 kV$_p$ with different lucite thickness with and without grid. Grid data: ratio 5, 30 lines/cm. Field size: 18×24 cm²

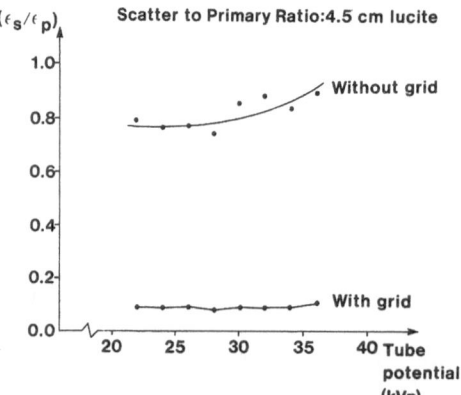

Fig. 11. Scatter to primary ratio as a function of tube potential without and with grid. Phantom thickness: 4.5 cm lucite. Grid data: ratio 5, 30 lines/cm. Field size: 18×24 cm²

Figure 11 shows that the scatter to primary ratio increases with increasing tube potential within the potential interval investigated (22–36 kV$_p$) when no grid is employed. Using a grid, the scatter to primary ratio is more or less constant with tube potential.

Different Methods of Reducing Scattered Radiation

There are several ways of reducing scatter and thus improving the mammographic image contrast. These include: compression, antiscatter grid, air gap, and scanning beam techniques. The scatter reductions obtained by stationary and moving grids, an air gap, and a scanning beam are compared in Table 1. The contrast for a 100-m-thick tin foil is shown as is the ratio of the scatter degradation factors with scatter reduction, SDF_g, and without scatter reduction, SDF (Morgan 1946; Bonenkamp and Hondius Boldingh 1959; Nielsen and Carlsson 1984).

The scatter degradation factor *(SDF)* is given by:

$$SDF=(1+\frac{\varepsilon_s}{\varepsilon_p})^{-1} \qquad (2)$$

The ratio SDF_g/SDF expresses how many times the contrast is enhanced due to reduction of scatter.

The calculated mean dose levels are also shown.

It can be seen from Table 1 that the most effective method for reduction of scattered radiation is the scanning beam technique. A stationary grid gives a slightly better scatter reduction than a moving one. The contrast with a moving grid is better than with a stationary one. The reason for this is partly due to filtration of the primary spectrum in the aluminum interspace of the stationary grid. The moving grid gives less filtration of the primary spectrum, because it has paper as interspace material. It can also be seen that there is better contrast with the magnification technique than with a grid. This is due to the smaller

Table 1. Comparison of methods for reducing the scattered radiation obtained with a 4-cm lucite phantom at 25 kV$_p$ tube potential. Field size: 18 × 24 cm². Stationary grid: ratio 3.5, 80 lines/cm, aluminum interspace material. Moving grid: ratio 5, 30 lines cm, paper interspace material. Developer temperature, 38° C

Mammographic technique	$\frac{\varepsilon_s}{\varepsilon_p}$	Contrast 0.1 mm Sn	Mean dose (mGy) normalized to optical density 1.2	$\frac{SDF_g}{SDF}$
Without scatter reduction	0.54	0.16	0.68	1.00
Moving grid	0.21	0.21	2.61	1.27
Stationary grid	0.16	0.19	2.98	1.33
Air gap 25 cm Lanex medium	0.13	0.24	1.62	1.36
Air gap 25 cm Lanex fine	0.13	0.24	3.98	1.36
Scanning beam data from Yester et al. (1981)	0.03	–	–	1.50

Table 2. Comparison of scatter to primary ratios obtained on a patient at 32 kV$_p$ tube potential. Field size: 18 × 24 cm^2. Grid data: ratio 5, 30 lines/cm

Method	Scatter to primary ratio $\varepsilon_s/\varepsilon_p$
No compression	1.6
With compression	0.7
With compression and grid	0.1

$\varepsilon_s/\varepsilon_p$ ratio and the reduced filtering of the primary photon spectrum in air than in the interspace and cover materials for a grid.

Note: The $\varepsilon_s/\varepsilon_p$ ratio for the moving grid in Table 1 is higher than that shown in Fig. 10. The reason for this is that with a grid or other scatter-reducing method, the measured optical density behind the lead beam stop is close to the optical density due to film fog. Because the film fog is subtracted from the optical density behind the lead beam stop, the accuracy of the measuring technique will be low and sensitive to changes in film fog and development conditions. The measurements in Fig. 10 and Table 1 for the moving grid are made on different occasions, giving low accuracy, while the data in Table 1 are made in one series, therefore giving correct values, relatively. The ratio of the scatter degradation factors *(SDF$_g$/SDF)* can be seen to be largest when the scanning beam technique is used or with an air gap. The scatter degradation ratio only considers the effect of scatter on contrast, while the measured contrast also incorporates the effect of the primary spectrum.

Compared with the no-grid technique, the mean dose levels with a grid can be seen to be increased by approximately a factor of 3–4. Stationary grids with aluminum interspaces give higher mean doses than those with paper interspaces. This can be expected from the different interspace materials. The air gap technique gives higher mean dose levels than the standard technique, because the object is moved closer to the X-ray tube. The air gap technique (magnification technique) also has a smaller field of view, which means that a smaller volume of the breast is irradiated. Depending on the volume imaged, the energy imparted to the breast may in fact be reduced using the magnification technique.

In Table 2, the effect of compression can be seen. The scatter to primary ratio was obtained on a patient with a lead beam stop. The measurements were carried out with and without compression and with both compression and grid.

Compression reduces the scattered radiation by a factor of 2, and when a grid is also used the $\varepsilon_s/\varepsilon_p$ ratio becomes very low.

Measurements of Absorbed Dose

Several authors have discussed dose measurements in mammography (Jennings et al. 1981; Beaman and Lillicrap 1983; Stanton et al. 1984). The average glandular dose has been assumed to be the best characterization of the radiation risk (Stanton et al. 1984).

The comparison of absorbed doses from different mammographic techniques is difficult to evaluate from measurements on patients because of the great variations in breast thickness and density. A study was made to measure the relative variation of absorbed dose in 80 women chosen on an arbitrary screening day. Values for milliampere second were recorded continuously with a constant tube potential of 25 kV$_p$. For the same film optical density, a spread in mAs values from 25 to 190 mAs was found. Due to this very large spread in mAs values, we find it less meaningful to compare absorbed doses for different techniques using patient measurements. To use one and the same patient for such a purpose would mean an unacceptably high dose to that individual. We have therefore chosen to use a phantom in comparing the absorbed doses from different techniques.

Because of the difficulties in determining the average glandular dose, we have used the mean dose to the phantom, calculating it from depth dose measurements using thermoluminescence dosimetry (TLD). Lithium fluoride (LiF) dosimeters 0.8 mm thick were placed in the phantom from top to bottom at 1-cm intervals. Measurements were obtained made for three different tube potentials: 25, 28, and 32 kV_p. The results are shown in Fig. 12, the depth doses being normalized to a total optical density of 1.2.

Figure 12 shows that when the tube potential is increased from 25 to 28 kV_p, the skin dose is reduced by approximately 30% and the ratio of entrance and exit doses from 42% to 34%.

From the depth dose curves in Fig. 12 the mean dose at the different kV_p:s was calculated. The results are shown in Fig. 13.

From Figs. 12 and 13, it can be seen that if the risk is considered to be best characterized by the mean dose, it is greatly overestimated by the entrance dose and underestimated by the midline dose.

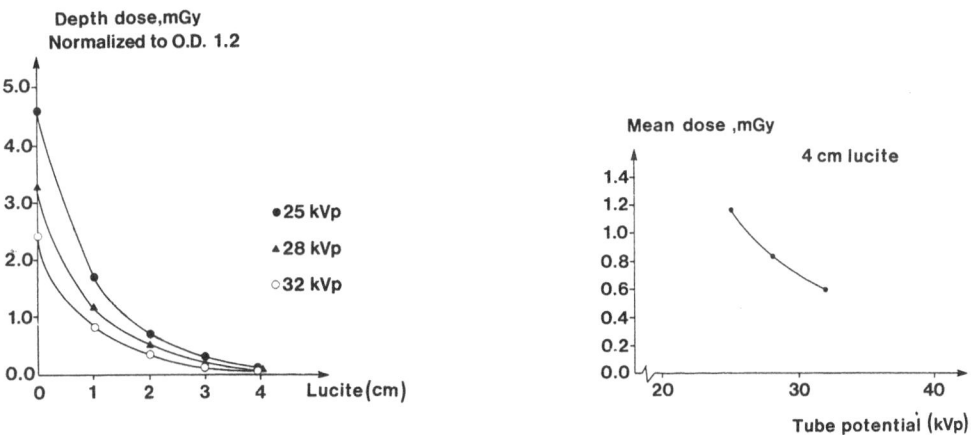

Fig. 12 *(left).* Depth dose measured with TLD-LiF dosimetry for a 4-cm phantom at 25, 28, and 32 kV_p

Fig. 13 *(right).* Mean dose as a function of tube potential for a 4-cm lucite phantom

Conclusions

From a comparison of simulated spectra of Mo anode/Mo filter tubes with W anode/Pd filter tubes behind 4 cm lucite, W tubes have more "high"-energy photons than Mo tubes. We therefore consider it unlikely that the contrast of W/Pd tubes can compete with Mo/Mo tubes at the same tube potential, although this has been reported, e.g., by Beaman et al. 1983 and McDonagh et al. 1984. In our opinion, the dose reduction found using W/Pd tubes is probably due to the fact that their mean energy is higher than for Mo/Mo tubes.

Table 3. Comparison of contrast and mean dose at 25 kV$_p$ and 28 kV$_p$ using a moving grid, a stationary grid, or no grid. Stationary grid: ratio 3.5, 80 lines/cm. Moving grid: ratio 5, 30 lines/cm. Developer temperature, 38° C

Mammographic technique	25 kV$_p$		28 kV$_p$	
	Contrast 0.1 mm Sn	Mean dose mGy	Contrast 0.1 mm Sn	Mean dose mGy
No grid	0.16	0.68	0.16	0.48
Moving grid paper interspace	0.22	2.61	0.18	1.54
Stationary grid Al interspace	0.20	2.98	0.20	1.60

In the standard mammographic technique, the magnification is so small that the factor limiting spatial resolution is normally determined by the fluorescent screen. Differences can be observed in images obtained using 0.3×0.3 mm^2 and 0.6×0.6 mm^2 foci.

With the standard technique the contrast is decreased mainly by scattered radiation, but it also decreases with increasing tube potential. The gain in contrast when the developer temperature is increased above 32° C is small and is not visible in phantom images.

When the mammographic magnification technique is used, the size of the focal spot is normally the factor limiting the spatial resolution. For a magnification of 2.2 and a focal spot size of 0.1×0.1 mm^2, the limiting factor is the fluorescent screen. The small loadability of this minute focal spot makes it necessary to use fluorescent screens faster than standard ones, thus making the screen the factor limiting the spatial resolution.

For the magnification technique, contrast is limited mainly by the tube potential. In practice, the lowest possible tube potential is approximately 25 kV$_p$.

Provided film development conditions have been optimized, scattered radiation is the main source of impaired contrast in mammography. With standard geometry, the best way to reduce scatter is to use the scanning beam technique. Although there are some prototype units working, this method is not yet in general clinical use. As in other radiographic examinations, use of a grid is the most practical way of reducing scatter in mammography. The severe technical problems arising in the development of optimized grids for mammography are due to the low photon energy involved.

The choice of tube potential is critical. Increasing the tube potential means a decrease in mean dose but at the same time reduces the contrast. In Table 3, a comparison of the parameters contrast and mean dose is made at 25 and 28 kV$_p$. From this table, the decrease in mean dose is clearly seen, while the improvement in contrast can only be said to be significant with a moving grid. The difference in mean dose between the two types of grid is greatest at 25 kV$_p$, at which potential the aluminum interspace of the stationary grid gives a higher attenuation than the paper interspace of the moving grid.

Our aim in this work has been to point out possible factors influencing image quality in mammography with the techniques available today, and how to optimize image quality. It has not been to minimize the dose. However, the absorbed doses registered in what we believe to be optimized standard and magnification techniques are so small that they are both acceptable and justifiable in relation to the benefit to the patient from the procedure. It should be pointed out that low image quality often also implies high absorbed doses.

In conclusion: we have found the optimized standard mammographic technique to be achieved under the following conditions: 25 kV$_p$, 0.6×0.6 mm^2 focal spot, film-focus distance 500 mm, antiscatter grid, developing temperature 37° C, and 4 min total processing time with the screen-film system we have used. If a magnification ratio of 2:1 is desired, a 0.1×0.1 mm^2 focal spot is mandatory. With this technique, it is necessary to use a faster screen-film system than that used in standard mammography.

References

Arnold BA, Eisenberg H, Bjarngard BE (1979) Magnification mammography: a low-dose technique. Radiology 131:743

Barnes GT, Brezovich IA (1978) The intensity of scattered radiation in mammography. Radiology 126:243

Basset LW, Arnold BA, Borger D, Eisenberg HG, Gold RH, Mahn GR, Holland WP (1981) Reduced-dose magnification mammography. Radiology 141:665

Beaman SA, Lillicrap SC (1982) Optimum x-ray spectra for mammography. Phys Med Biol 27:1209

Beaman S, Lillicrap SC, Price JL (1983) Tungsten anode tubes with k-edge filters for mammography. Brit J Radiol 56:721

Birch R, Marshall M, Ardran GM (1979) Catalogue of spectral data for diagnostic X-rays. The Hospital Physicists' Association Scientific Report Series, vol 30

Bonenkamp JG, Hondius Boldingh W (1959) Quality and choice of Potter Bucky grids. Acta Radiol 51:479

Dance DR, Day GJ (1984) The computation of scatter in mammography by Monte Carlo methods. Phys Med Biol 29:237

DeSmet AA, Fritz SL, Tempelton AW (1982) Direct radiographic magnification: evaluation of three microfocus x-ray tubes. Am J Radiol 138:139

Doi K, Imhof H (1977) Noise reduction by radiographic magnification. Radiology 122:479

Egan RL, McSweeney MB, Sewell CW (1980) Intramammary calcifications without an associated mass in benign and malignant disease. Radiology 137:1

Feig SA (1983) Assessment of hypothetical risk from mammography and evaluation of the potential benefit. Radiol Clin North Am 21:173

Friedrich M (1978) Neuere Entwicklungstendenzen der Mammographie-Technik: Die Raster-Mammographie. Fortschr Röntgenstr 128:207

Friedrich M, Weskamp P (1976) Bildgütefaktoren bei der Filmmammographie. Fortschr Röntgenstr 125:269

Gould RG, Genant HK (1981) Quantitative and qualitative comparison of two microfocus-tube imaging systems. Radiology 138:195

Hammerstein GR, Miller DW, White DR et al. (1979) Absorbed radiation dose in mammography. Radiology 130:485

Haus AG (1984) Screen-film update, X-ray units, breast compression, grids, screen-film characteristics and radiation dose. Medical Imaging and Instrumentation 84. Prac Spie Vol 486

ICRP 26, Publication 26 (1977) Recommendations of the International Commission on Radiological Protection. Ann ICRP 1, 3

Jennings RJ, Fewell TR (1979) Filters – photon energy control and patient exposure. In: Logan WW, Munty EP (eds) Reduced dose mammography. Masson, New York, p 211

Jennings RJ, Eastgate RJ, Siedband MP, Ergun DL (1981) Optimal x-ray spectra for screen-film mammography. Med Phys 8:629

King MA, Barnes GT, Yester MV (1979) A mammographic scanning multiple slit assembly: design considerations and preliminary results. In: Logan WW, Muntz EP (eds) Reduced dose mammography. Masson, New York

Lammers W, Kuhn H (1979) Improved image quality in mammography by means of scattered radiation grids. Siemens Electro-medica

Lester RG (1977) Risk versus benefit in mammography. Radiology 124:1

McDonagh CP, Leake JL, Beaman SA (1984) Optimum x-ray spectra for mammography: choice of K-filters for tungsten anode tubes. Phys Med Biol 29:249

Morgan RH (1946) An analysis of the physical factors controlling the diagnostic quality of roentgen images. Part III. Contrast and the intensity distribution function of a roentgen image. Am J Roentgenol 55: 67

Muntz EP (1979a) Analysis of the significance of scattered radiation in reduced dose mammography, including magnification effects, scatter suppression, and detector blurring. Med Phys 6: 110

Muntz EP (1979b) Relative carcinogenic effects of different mammography techniques. Med Phys 6: 205

NCRP Report 66 (1980) Mammography. National Council on Radiation Protection and Measurements, Washington DC

Nielsen B, Carlsson CA (1984) Energy imparted to fluorescent screens from primary and scattered radiation. Variations with atomic composition and screen thickness. Phys Med Biol 29: 315

O'Foghludha F, Johnson GA (1981) Voltage waveform effects on output and penetration of W- and Mo-anode mammographic tubes. Phys Med Biol 26: 291

Rossmann K (1964) Measurement of the modulation transfer function of radiographic systems containing fluorescent screens. Phys Med Biol 9: 551

Stanton L, Villafana T, Day JL et al. (1984) Dose evaluation in mammography. Radiology 150: 577

Wagner RF, Barnes GT, Askins BS (1980) Effect of reduced scatter on radiographic information content and patient exposure: a quantitative demonstration. Med Phys 7: 13

Yester MV, Barnes GT, King MA (1981) Experimental measurements of the scatter reduction obtained in mammography with scanning multiple slit assembly. Med Phys 8: 158

Clinical Considerations in Selection of Dedicated Mammography Units

S. A. Feig, B. M. Galkin, and H. D. Muir

Department of Radiology, Thomas Jefferson University Hospital, Philadelphia, PA 191107, USA

Several aspects of dedicated mammography units are better evaluated by means of patient examinations than by studies on breast phantoms. These include the ability to (1) achieve optimal breast compression and positioning, (2) use short exposure times to minimize the chance of motion unsharpness, (3) obtain proper exposure by means of a phototimer or manual exposure settings, and (4) accommodate different size breasts.

Breast Compression and Positioning

Both the compression plate and the table on which the cassette rests should be straight on the side facing the patient rather than curved. Those which are convex to fit the chest wall curvature for the craniocaudal view may prevent the film from getting sufficiently close to the chest wall for the oblique view in some patients.

The compression plate should also be completely parallel to the surface of the film. If there is significant posterior sloping of the device, decreased compression and underpenetration of the back of the breast will occur.

The posterior aspect of the compression device should be bent upwards at a 90° angle for 3-4 cm to (1) provide structural strength so that the plastic will not fracture during vigorous compression, (2) push back the axillary fat fold from the lateral aspect of the breast on the craniocaudal view, and (3) prevent the back of the breast from slipping out from under the device.

Some dedicated units come with several compression devices of different sizes to match the size of the breast being examined. This is a useful feature because if the compression device is substantially larger than the breast, it will interfere with the technologist's hand being placed under the device to position the breast, smooth out the skin folds, and pull the breast from the chest wall.

Most compression plates are made of plastic, usually of 1-4 mm thickness. Thicker plates may require increased exposure time unless they result in greater compression.

Some units employ a motorized precompression device controlled by a foot switch. This leaves the operator's hands free for positioning the patient. When this device is used, there should be provision for manual fine tuning to provide final compression after the motorized action fixes the breast in position. The force of precompression can be chosen with a knob. When a preset force is reached, an electromagnetic clutch insures that this value is not exceeded so that excessive pressure is not applied.

In other units, the compression pad is lowered manually. However, regardless of the type of device employed, it must provide strong, steady compression without slippage. In some units, this may be a problem in firm breasts.

Recent Results in Cancer Research. Vol 105
© Springer-Verlag Berlin · Heidelberg 1987

During positioning, film bags or cassettes are held to the mammography machine table top by a clamping device. The types of clamps employed on some units will firmly secure the film bags or cassettes while others may permit them to slip.

The tube should be capable of positioning at 45° from the vertical for the standard oblique view, at 30° or 60° for oblique view positioning in some short, stocky or tall, thin patients, and at other angles for tangential views.

Short Exposure Times

The length of exposure is an extremely important feature which is frequently overlooked in selecting a mammographic unit. There are significant differences in exposure times among currently available mammographic units. Motion unsharpness may begin to appear on some films when exposure times exceed 1 s and will become a significant problem with exposure times of 2 s or more. With inadequate compression, considerable motion unsharpness can be seen even with exposure times of 0.2 s (National Council on Radiation Protection and Measurements 1986).

Patients whose breasts are larger, less compressible, or more fibroglandular and those where grid and magnification studies are performed will require longer exposure times than other patients. Grid and magnification studies both require a higher milliampere second (mAs) value since less scattered radiation will reach the film (Stanton and Logan 1979; Sickles 1982; Egan et al. 1983). Magnification studies may also be more susceptible to motion unsharpness since they require smaller focal spot tubes which have a lower milliampere (mA) output than the larger focal spot tubes used in conventional mammography (Haus et al. 1979).

In many cases, motion unsharpness may be due to human factors as well as equipment. Motion unsharpness can be minimized if as much compression is applied as can be comfortably tolerated by the patient. The technologist should explain to her slowly, carefully, and calmly that vigorous compression is necessary to obtain a study which provides the most information, that such compression will be applied only briefly, and that it will be no more uncomfortable than the application of a blood pressure cuff. If the patient is told beforehand to be prepared to hold her breath, she will be able to do so better than if she were not previously alerted.

Besides resulting in motion unsharpness, long exposure times may also cause either decreased optical density of the film or increased dose due to reciprocity law failure. At long exposure times, the density is less than expected from the product of the X-ray beam intensity and the time of exposure. Thus, there is loss of film speed (Arnold et al. 1978; Bencomo and Haus 1978; Haus et al. 1979).

A higher generator output, specified in mA units, will allow shorter exposure times. One must, however, take care in comparing the exposure times of different units on the basis of the mA output stated in the manufacturer's literature since, for a given X-ray mammography unit, the mA output will vary according to kVp, focal spot size, and length of exposure.

Because of generator limitations, the maximum allowable mA output may be reduced as the kVp is raised. For most mammography units, the mA output at 32 kVp will be about 25% less than at 25 kVp.

The maximum mA output will also be limited by focal spot size. For one dedicated unit where 0.1-, 0.3-, and 0.6-mm focal spot sizes are available, the output for each was 25, 100, and 200 mA respectively.

One mammography unit is able to perform magnification work by means of a single filament which is electronically altered to change the size of the focal spot from 0.5 to 0.2 mm. However, the mA output from such a 0.5-mm focal spot is only 50% that of the 0.6-mm focal spot previously used by this manufacturer. Thus, the use of a variable (electron bias) focal spot for nonmagnified work could result in longer exposure times than a system employing two separate filaments.

The mA output provided in a tube rating is given at cold or ambient anode temperature. Besides the tube rating, the mA output may also be influenced by the heat storage capacity of the anode. If the anode is hot from repeated use, the mA output of a tube with a lower heat storage capacity might be less than that of a tube with a higher heat storage capacity. This parameter will also vary among dedicated mammography units.

Differences in exposure times between mammography units may result not only from mA output, but also from differences in the focal spot-film distance (FFD). A machine with a longer FFD will require a higher mAS to achieve the same amount of exposure according to the inverse square law. For example, for an FFD of 65 cm the required mAS would be 17% $[(65/60)^2]$ more than for an FFD of 60 cm and 40% $[(65/55)^2]$ more than for an FFD of 55 cm. Most newer mammography units have an FFD of 50 cm or more. One unit we tested was capable of operating a four positions from 50 to 65 cm.

The mA output will also depend on the length of exposure since there will be a decrease in mA output during the course of any exposure, i. e., a higher mAs will result in lower average mA output.

Proper Exposure

If phototiming is provided, the phototimer cell (ionization chamber) will be contained in the film-support table top. Proper positioning of the phototimer is important. If the phototimer is not entirely covered by breast tissue, films will be underexposed. Most dedicated mammography units have two or three photocell locations, each at a different distance from the edge of the film support, to which the phototimer can be shifted. For small breasts, the phototimer location closest to the chest should be used for all views. The distance of this phototimer position from the edge of the film tray will differ among dedicated mammography units. The closer it is to the tray edge and the smaller the phototimer cell, the less likely will be the possibility of underexposure in small breasts. For medium- and large-size breasts, the phototimer position closest to the chest wall should also be used for the lateral oblique view since placement of the phototimer under the pectoralis will insure proper exposure of the denser posterior tissues. In these size breasts, the phototimer should be placed under the mid-breast for the craniocaudal view to ensure representative thickness and density.

Among dedicated mammography units, there are differences in the flexibility of choices allowed for selection of kVp, mA, or mAs and density settings. Within the 22- to 34-kVp range used for screen-film studies, some units allow 12 steps of 1 kVp each whereas other units may permit only 5 steps of 2 or 3 kVp each. When manual timing is used, one unit may offer 28-mAs steps from 4 to 800 mAs while another provides 13 steps from 0.2 to 4.0 s. The density control setting has 11 steps (-5 to $+5$) of 20% each in one unit, but three steps (-1, 0, $+1$) of 25% each in another. In addition, this first unit has a film density selector which may used to further adjust the overall level of phototimer density settings for different screen-film combinations or for nongrid, grid, or magnification studies. Availability of multiple phototimer density settings can be useful in obtaining consistently satisfactory film densities despite the difference in compressed breast thickness and kVp technique (Niklason et al. 1985).

Accommodation of Different Size Breasts

Although most patient's breasts can be accommodated on an 18 × 24-cm-size film, in our practice, approximately 20% of patients require a 24 × 30-cm film to include the axillary tail. Some units may not accommodate a 24 × 30-cm cassette or vacuum bag or may not secure them firmly so that they may move during exposure.

At present, a 24 × 30-cm grid is not commercially available on all mammography units. In one unit, when this larger size grid is placed in position, the grid extends several centimeters beyond the edge of the phototimer. Since the photocell is no longer directly under the pectoralis muscle on the oblique view, underexposure of the deeper tissues may result.

Mammography units may allow collimation by providing a set of fixed-size diaphragms which fit into the cone or a continuously adjustable diaphragm which provides even better tailored collimation. Many units have a light localizer to insure proper centering of the breast and the collimator.

User Considerations

All accessories such as grid, magnification platform, compression device, and cone should be easily fitted on, firmly locked in place, and easily removed from the mammography machine. The unit should be designed with patient comfort in mind. The patient's body should not be in contact with rough or sharp edges or corners. In addition, a plastic edge will feel less cold to the skin than a metal one. With regard to these user considerations, some mammography units are better designed than others.

References

Arnold BA, Eisenberg H, Bjärngard BE (1978) Measurement of reciprocity law failure in green-sensitivity x-ray films. Radiology 126: 493–498

Bencomo J, Haus AG (1978) The effect of reciprocity law failure when determining the characteristic curve for screen-film systems. Med Phys 5: 322–323

Egan RL, McSweeney MB, Sprawls P (1983) Grids in mammography. Radiology 146: 359–362

Haus AG, Paulus DD, Dodd GD, et al. (1979) Magnification mammography: evaluation of screen-film and xeroradiographic techniques. Radiology 133: 223–226

National Council on Radiation Protection and Measurements (1986) Mammography – a user's guide. Bethesda, p 21 (NCRP Report No 85)

Niklason LT, Barnes GT, Rubin E (1985) Mammography phototimer technique chart. Radiology 157: 539–540

Sickles EA (1982) Magnification mammography. In: Bassett LW, Gold RH (eds) Mammography, thermography and ultrasound in breast cancer detection. Grune and Stratton, New York, pp 87–94

Stanton L, Logan WW (1979) Mammography with magnification and grids: detail visibility and dose measurements. In: Logan WW, Muntz EP (eds) Reduced dose mammography. Masson, New York, pp 259–264

The Role of Magnification Technique in Modern Mammography

E. A. Sickles

Department of Radiology, Breast Imaging Section, University of California School of Medicine, San Francisco, CA 94143, USA

Magnification mammography is an adjunct to conventional mammographic technique. It produces fine-detail breast images containing additional anatomic information that may prove useful in refining mammographic diagnosis, especially in cases where conventional imaging demonstrates uncertain or equivocal findings.

Equipment Requirements

Conventional mammography is done with the breast directly in contact with the X-ray film cassette, producing essentially life-size images. Geometric blurring of conventional mammograms is kept to a minimum by vigorous breast compression, bringing areas of abnormality as close as possible to the film. Magnification technique, on the other hand, interposes an air gap between breast and film, so that the projected radiographic image is enlarged. Because of the resultant increase in imaging distance, one must use higher kVp, faster film, longer exposures, or a combination of these factors to produce magnification mammograms (Sickles 1984).

Magnification technique requires the use of an X-ray tube that has a very small focal spot, to render inconsequential the considerable unsharpness that otherwise would accompany geometric image enlargement. Laboratory evidence suggests that the largest acceptable focal spot size for 1.5 X magnification mammography is 0.3 mm in greatest diameter (Muntz and Logan 1979), a specification met by some but not all dedicated mammography units currently being promoted to have magnification capability. Greater amounts of magnification require even smaller focal spots. It is crucial to realize that this 0.3-mm limit refers to actual (measured) focal spot size, not the (nominal) size claimed by the equipment manufacturer. Unfortunately, there often is a difference between these two sizes, measured size typically being almost twice as large. This suggests that 1.5 X magnification imaging will always be successful with focal spots nominally 0.1 mm in size or smaller, but that nominal 0.2-mm focal spots may or may not prove adequate and that even larger focal spots will usually produce disappointing clinical results. However, because nominal focal spot size is such an unreliable indicator of imaging performance, it is preferable for prospective buyers of magnification mammography equipment to insist on purchase specifications that guarantee measured focal spot size. It is also important for magnification mammography equipment to permit vigorous breast compression, primarily because the relatively long exposure times used for magnification imaging provide an increased opportunity for image blurring due to motion unsharpness.

Laboratory Results

The superior image quality of magnification mammograms has been studied extensively in the laboratory (Sickles et al. 1977; Haus et al. 1979). Provided that an appropriately small focal spot is used for the selected degree of magnification, resolution is increased and effective system noise is reduced with magnification technique, producing sharper, more detailed images. These findings have been documented qualitatively by imaging wire mesh and plastic bead test objects and quantitatively by the measurement of modulation transfer functions (MTF) and Wiener spectra. Theoretically, magnification technique should also result in increased image contrast, due to air-gap elimination of scattered radiation. However, the relatively small air gaps used in clinical practice actually result in very little contrast enhancement, and frequently this is offset by the higher kVp often required to produce properly exposed images.

The additional exposure requirements of magnification imaging can be satisfied entirely by very fast screens and films, resulting in doses similar to or even lower than conventional mammography (Arnold et al. 1979; Sickles 1979; Bassett et al. 1981). However, the increased speed of the recording systems used in these low-dose magnification techniques generally degrades overall image quality to a clinically unacceptable degree. As a result, almost all current magnification techniques impart higher doses than conventional mammography.

Clinical Experience

The most extensive published clinical experience with magnification mammography is that of Sickles et al. (1977; 1979; 1980). This prospective controlled clinical trial involved 750 selected patients, approximately equal numbers of whom were studied with screen-film mammography and xeromammography. For each patient, a single additional 1.5X magnification mammogram was obtained immediately after interpretation of a full conventional mammography examination. The combination of conventional and magnification images then was reinterpreted to determine the frequency and extent of any changes in diagnostic impression.

There were no meaningful differences in results for screen-film versus xeroradiographic technique. However, the 1.5X magnification mammograms almost always produced sharper, more detailed images than their conventional 1X counterparts. Additional anatomic information frequently was available on the magnification images, including improved visualization of subtle areas of architectural distortion, the margins of breast masses, and the shape, number, and distribution of breast calcifications.

Occasionally, magnification mammography detected a small breast carcinoma that had been completely missed on the entire conventional examination, but by far the major impact of magnification technique was to permit more precise mammographic diagnosis of lesions otherwise demonstrating only equivocal radiographic findings. In some instances the increased detail of the magnification images permitted the mammographic diagnosis of carcinoma to be made with confidence where at best it could be suspected on the conventional examination. In an even greater number of cases, the ability of magnification mammography to define the smooth, sharp borders of a benign mass or the round and oval shapes of tiny benign calcifications removed a substantial amount of the suspicion of malignancy that had been raised on conventional films. Overall, in the selected patient population studied, approximately 70% of the cases initially read as equivocal for

Table 1. Mammographic interpretations (750 patients)

Conventional mammography	Conventional + magnification mammography
227 benign	201 benign 19 equivocal 7 malignant
496 equivocal	297 benign 151 equivocal 48 malignant
27 malignant	27 malignant

Table 2. Radiologic-pathologic correlations (251 patients)

Mammographic diagnosis		Pathologic diagnosis	
Conventional	Conventional + magnification		
56 benign	38 benign 12 equivocal 6 malignant	36 benign 9 benign 6 malignant	2 malignant 3 malignant
168 equivocal	57 benign 63 equivocal 48 malignant	57 benign 44 benign 1 benign	19 malignant 47 malignant
27 malignant	27 malignant	27 malignant	

malignancy were interpreted as either benign or malignant after viewing the additional magnification mammogram (Table 1).

Biopsy was done on approximately one-third of the study patients within 1 month of examination, and radiographic-pathologic correlation showed a striking increase in diagnostic accuracy for magnification technique (Table 2). This was especially true among patients whose conventional mammograms were given equivocal interpretations. Of the 48 cases read as frankly malignant because of the additional magnification mammogram, only one interpretation proved to be in error; and all 57 of the cases read as benign after magnification mammography were indeed benign at biopsy. Furthermore, careful follow-up was done on those study patients not undergoing biopsy whose mammographic diagnoses were changed from equivocal to benign as a result of magnification images. All of these patients now have been observed for more than 5 years, and none have developed cancer in or adjacent to the area where conventional mammograms initially suggested some suspicion of malignancy.

The increased diagnostic accuracy of magnification mammography translates readily into improved patient management. Magnification imaging provides the impetus for more prompt biopsy of some cancers, either because it detects nonpalpable malignant lesions that were not even suspected on conventional mammograms, or because it adds sufficient suspicion of malignancy to an otherwise equivocal lesion as to convince a reluctant patient or surgeon to choose biopsy in favor of clinical observation. However, a much more substantial effect of magnification mammography on patient management is the reduction in the number of biopsies for lesions that prove to be benign. This occurs when magnification mammograms substantially reduce or completely eliminate the suspicion of malignancy that had been indicated by conventional 1X examination. Most of these patients are observed clinically and have repeat magnification mammography examinations instead of undergoing biopsy. In my own experience I have followed more than 1000 such cases over multiple-year intervals, and none of the initially suspicious lesions have proved to be malignant.

Many manufacturers of mammography equipment have been supplying imaging systems with magnification capability for several years, and it is reasonable to assume that there now has been widespread clinical experience with the technique. Additional controlled clinical studies have not been published, but several distinguished breast imaging experts have reported considerable anecdotal experience supporting the clinical utility of magnification mammography (Logan 1977; Bassett et al. 1981; Logan 1983; Paulus et al. 1981; Tabar 1984). As a result, the technique is generally accepted as a useful breast imaging tool.

Practical Applications

The most clearly established role of magnification mammography is as an adjunct to conventional mammography when the initial study is interpreted as equivocal for malignancy. However, additional indications for magnification technique abound.

1. When a nonpalpable yet suspicious lesion is seen on only one of the two standard projections with conventional mammography, magnification imaging may clearly demonstrate the abnormality on the other view, thereby permitting prompt radiographic localization for biopsy. All too often, without the use of magnification the only alternative is to wait for the lesion to grow, until it eventually gets biopsied either because it becomes palpable or visible on more than one standard mammographic view.
2. Sometimes, conventional mammograms show barely perceptible or extremely subtle findings that are too innocuous to suggest malignancy in and of themselves. Magnification technique can prove immensely valuable in these situations by indicating more definitively the presence of truly suspicious lesions, prompting earlier biopsy of small breast cancers. This occurs most commonly when only two or three adjacent nondescript calcific particles are identified on conventional 1X images but magnification mammograms demonstrate a cluster of five or more suspicious microcalcifications.
3. Although additional conventional mammographic projections such as oblique views, tangential views, and spot films can provide new perspectives to better assess questionable radiographic findings (Gershon-Cohen et al. 1965; Buchanan and Jager 1978; Hall and Berenberg 1978; Kopans et al. 1983; Homer 1985), magnification technique also can be done using these alternative projections, offering the further advantage of increased image detail.
4. Finally, there even is an indication for magnification mammography when conventional imaging already indicates the presence of malignancy: not infrequently, otherwise unsuspected multicentric foci of tumor are identified only with magnification technique (Sickles and Weber 1985). Thus, for a specific patient, magnification mammography can be very useful in determining whether excisional biopsy and comprehensive radiation therapy indeed represent an acceptable alternative to mastectomy by more accurately delineating tumor size and extent.

Further Considerations

Despite the fact that magnification imaging frequently outperforms conventional 1X technique in many specific circumstances, magnification examinations are not recommended as a first-line procedure. Rather, one should rely on conventional mammography to identify abnormalities and then proceed to magnification exposures if additional information is needed to further characterize questionable or equivocal findings. Even in the selected series of difficult-to-evaluate patients illustrated in Table 1, magnification technique detected totally unsuspected cancers in only 1% of cases. In the average patient population, this yield would be much lower still.

Another valid concern limiting the general utilization of magnification mammography is that it imparts a radiation dose 1.5–4 times higher than standard 1X techniques (Sickles 1979; Haus et al. 1979). These higher doses are entirely acceptable for the one-time evaluation or periodic short-term follow-up of radiographically questionable lesions, for which the likelihood of malignancy is substantial. However, a complete examination of both breasts with magnification technique would require at least four higher-dose exposures, and twice as many as this for large-breasted women in order to include all the breast tissue on currently available recording systems. And since the general mammography patient population is heavily weighted with asymptomatic women in whom a very low yield of breast cancer is expected, it is much more prudent to use lower-dose conventional 1X mammography as the initial examination.

Conclusions

Magnification mammography is an invaluable breast imaging technique to supplement the occasionally inadequate information provided by conventional mammography. If utilized in appropriately selected patients it can be expected to substantially improve diagnostic accuracy and favorably affect management decisions. Radiologists interested in providing magnification mammography services must obtain the proper equipment, train their technical personnel to use it correctly, and develop the necessary expertise in interpreting fine-detail images of the breasts.

References

Arnold BA, Eisenberg H, Bjärngard BE (1979) Magnification mammography: a low-dose technique. Radiology 131: 743–749

Bassett LW, Arnold BA, Borger D, et al. (1981) Reduced dose magnification mammography. Radiology 141: 665–670

Buchanan JB, Jager RM (1978) Contact spot xeromammography in the early diagnosis of breast cancer. Am J Roentgenol 130: 1159–1162

Gershon-Cohen J, Berger SM, Delpino L (1965) Mammography: some remarks on techniques. Radiol Clin N Am 3: 389–401

Hall FM, Berenberg AL (1978) Selective use of the oblique projection in mammography. Am J Roentgenol 131: 465–468

Haus AG, Paulus DD, Dodd GD, et al. (1979) Magnification mammography: evaluation of screen-film and xeroradiographic techniques. Radiology 133: 223–226

Homer MJ (1985) Breast imaging: pitfalls, controversies, and some practical thoughts. Radiol Clin N Am 23: 459–472

Kopans DB, Meyer JE, Homer MJ et al. (1983) Dermal deposits mistaken for breast calcifications. Radiology 149: 592–594

Logan WW (1977) Overview of the radiologist's role in breast cancer detection. In: Logan WW (ed) Breast carcinoma: the radiologist's expanded role. Wiley, New York, pp 343–365

Logan WW (1983) Screen-film mammography: technique. In: Feig SA, McLelland R (eds) Breast carcinoma. Current diagnosis and treatment. Masson, New York, pp 141–160

Muntz EP, Logan WW (1979) Focal spot size and scatter suppression in magnification mammography. Am J Roentgenol 133: 453–459

Paulus DD, Lindell MM, Libshitz HI et al. (1981) Clinical evaluation of magnification mammography. Presented at annual meeting of Radiological Society of North America, Chicago

Sickles EA, Doi K, Genant HK (1977) Magnification film mammography: image quality and clinical studies. Radiology 125: 69–76

Sickles EA (1979) Microfocal spot magnification mammography using xeroradiographic and screen-film recording systems. Radiology 131: 599–607

Sickles EA (1980) Further experience with microfocal spot magnification mammography in the assessment of clustered breast microcalcifications. Radiology 137: 9–14

Sickles EA (1984) Dedicated mammography equipment. In: Syllabus for the categorical course on mammography. American College of Radiology, Chevy Chase, MD, pp 1–7

Sickles EA, Weber WN (1985) Magnification mammography to evaluate extent of breast cancer in women desiring alternative treatments to mastectomy. Radiology 157 (P): 174

Tabár L (1984) Microfocal spot magnification mammography. In: Brünner S, Langfeldt B, Andersen PE (eds) Early detection of breast cancer. Springer, Berlin Heidelberg New York Tokyo, pp 62–68

Imaging Capabilities and Dose Considerations of Different Mammographic Units

B. M. Galkin, S. A. Feig, P. Frasca, H. D. Muir, and R. Z. Soriano

Departments of Radiology and Orthopedic Surgery, Stein Research Center,
Thomas Jefferson University Hospital, 920 Chancellor Street, Philadelphia, PA 19107, USA

Introduction

Physicians who are planning to buy a new mammographic unit often find the selection difficult because the units from different manufacturers differ in important features which, theoretically, could affect image quality and patient dose. Moreover, there is a considerable range in the price of equipment from different manufacturers. The purpose of this study was to compare the diagnostic quality and patient dose for some state-of-the-art (1984) dedicated mammographic units.

Methods and Materials

Tests were conducted on the four mammographic units identified in Table 1. These were selected because they were available and because they differed in price by about a factor of 3.

The intent was to determine the effect of the mammographic unit itself, so all other factors that could influence image quality and patient dose were controlled. Therefore, the same cassette/screen combination and a single type of film were used for each comparative study. All films were developed in the same processor, which was subject to daily quality assurance checks.

Focal spot sizes and shapes were determined using the pinhole and star pattern methods. Exposure and beam quality (HVL in aluminum) were calculated from measurements made with a Radcal Model 10X5-6M chamber coupled to a Radcal 1015 X-ray monitor. Calibration of this system was traceable to the US National Bureau of Standards.

Two excised female breasts from different cadavers were used as phantoms to simulate clinical images. The breasts were kept in formalin between studies and the formalin was allowed to drain before the radiographs were taken. To maintain reproducible geometry each breast was sutured along the posterior margin so that the mammogram for one was a

Table 1. Mammographic units included in this study

Manufacturer	Model
CGR	Senographe 500 T
Elscint	MAM LS-3
Kramex	MX-43
Philips	Diagnost U-M

lateral projection and a craniocaudad projection for the other. A uniform amount of compression was applied for each mammogram using the compression plate supplied with each unit. The compressed thickness was approximately 5 cm for the lateral and 6 cm for the craniocaudad view.

Patient doses were calculated on the basis of exposure measurements for mammograms that were matched in overall density within limits imposed by extant exposure factors programmed into the units. Doses were calculated using the method described by Stanton (1984).

Subjective evaluation of the mammograms was made by querying over 100 radiologists who viewed the images which were displayed in a scientific exhibit at the 1984 Scientific Assembly and Annual Meeting of the Radiological Society of North America, Washington, DC (Galkin, Feig, Frasca et al. 1984). No attempt was made to determine the level of mammography expertise of those interviewed.

Results

Table 2 contains data on the effective focal spots for the four units. The tube in the Kramex unit contained only one (large) focal spot. Pinhole and star pattern images for the large focal spots are shown in Figs. 1 and 2.

Beam quality was measured at the tube potentials recommended by company representatives to image a 5-cm moderately glandular breast. The results are shown in Table 3. Since the intention was to evaluate the quality of the beams actually striking the patient, the HVLs were measured at the patient side of the compression plate located ~5 cm above the film holder.

Skin exposures for the different units were normalized to the lowest dose unit. The results are shown in Table 4.

Table 2. Focal spot measurements for different mammographic units

Mammographic unit	Small focal spot		Large focal spot	
	Effective size (mm)	Shape	Effective size (mm)	Shape
CGR	0.1 × 0.2	Oval	0.2 × 0.5	Bilinear
Elscint	0.1	Round	0.8	Annular
Kramex	None	–	0.4 × 0.7	Bilinear
Philips	0.2 × 0.3	Bilobed	0.4 × 0.7	Bilobed

Table 3. Beam quality for different mammographic units

Unit	Recommended kV[a]	Measured HVL mm Al
CGR	28	0.31
Elscint	24	0.24
Kramex	29	0.39
Philips	28	0.35

[a] Recommended by company representatives.

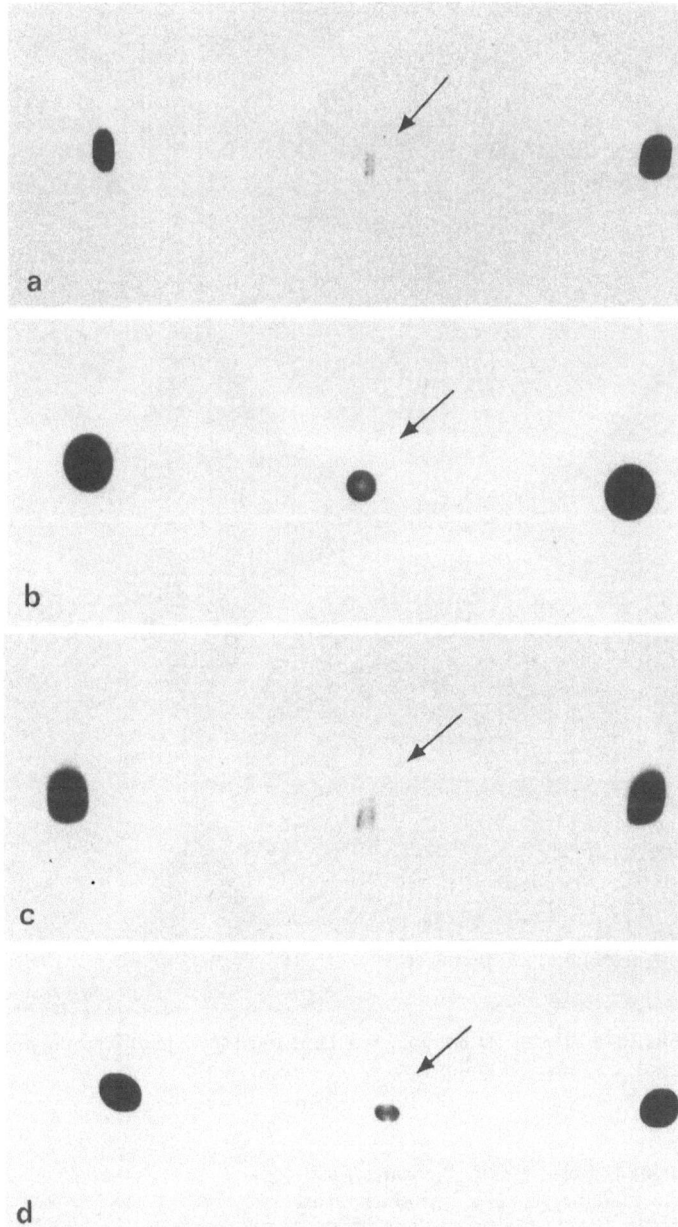

Fig. 1a–d. The *arrows* point to pinhole images of the large focal spots in different mammographic units. The *large spots on either side* are images of holes in the test tool used for alignment purposes and to measure the degree of magnification. **a** CGR; **b** Elscint; **c** Kramex; **d** Philips

Relative skin exposures for contact, grid, and magnified views for each unit are listed in Table 5.

Average glandular doses for a 6-cm-thick compressed breast using Kodak NMB film and a Min-R screen are shown in Table 6.

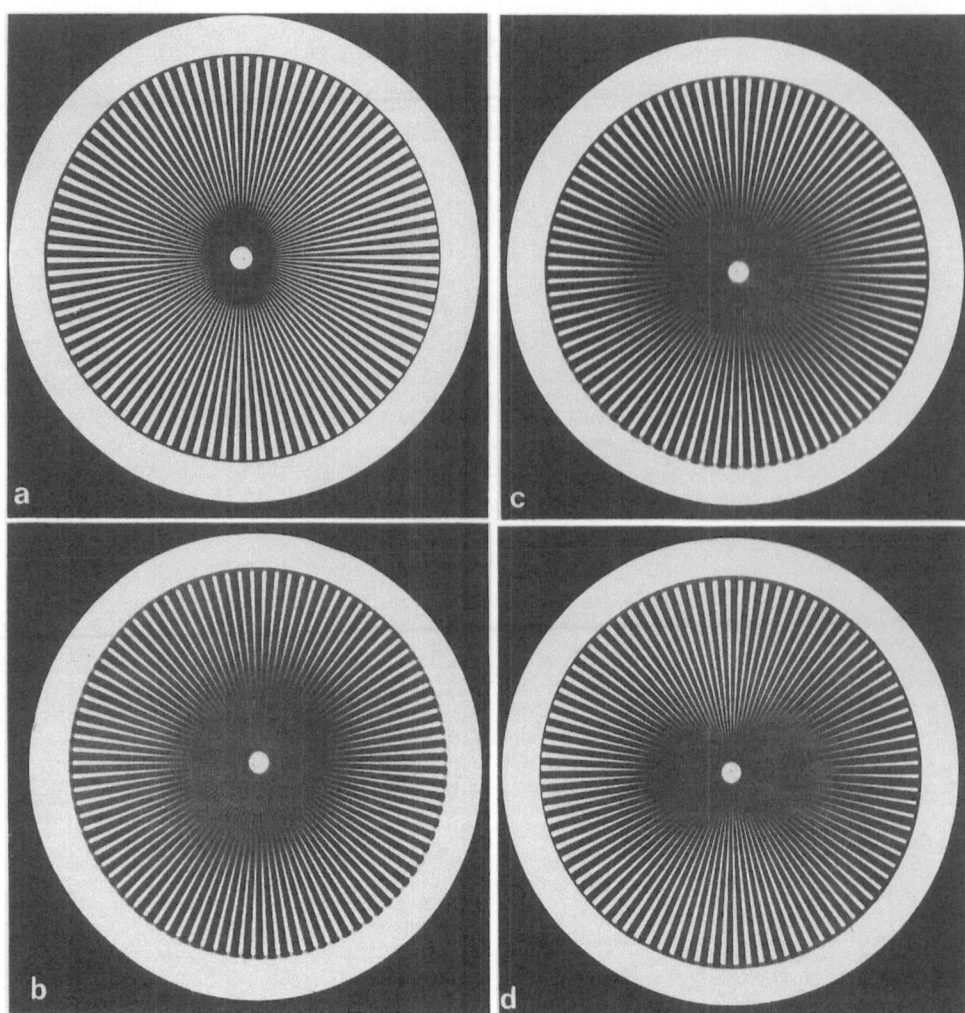

Fig. 2 a–d. 2° star pattern images of large focal spots in different mammographic units. **a** CGR; **b** El-scint; **c** Kramex; **d** Philips

Table 4. Relative skin exposures for a con-tact mammogram of a 5-cm-thick breast

Mammographic unit	Relative exposure
CGR	1.11
Elscint	1.00
Kramex	1.21
Philips	1.16

Table 5. Relative skin exposures for different mammographic techniques

View	Relative exposure			
Unit:	CGR	Elscint	Philips	Kramex
Contact	1.0	1.0	1.0	1.0
Grid	2.0	1.7	1.6	None
Magnified	8.5	1.8	3.1	None
degree	~2.0×	~1.5×	~1.75×	–

Table 6. Average glandular dose for a 6-cm-thick breast (Min R Screen/NMB Film)

	mad
CGR	88
Elscint	73
Kramex	109
Philips	99

Discussion

The tables and figures show sizable differences in focal spot dimensions and shapes, and in half-value layers for the different mammographic units. Theoretically, these differences should be reflected in the quality of the mammograms.

A study was conducted to test this theory. Using one of the excised breasts as a phantom, four unlabeled lateral contact mammograms, one from each unit, were matched for density whithin the limits explained above. The mammograms were displayed side-by-side on a view box. Directly beneath them but in a different order were four similarly matched unlabeled contact craniocaudad mammograms of the other breast. The physicians were asked to grade the images in each row. The overwhelming majority said there was no significant difference in the diagnostic quality of the images in each group and very few were able to match images from the same units.

The dosage data for this part of the study (Table 4) appear to suggest that patient doses are related to the mammographic units. However, this conclusion is premature since the doses were determined for mammograms that were not exactly matched for density as explained previously.

In another test of the theory, lateral contact, grid, and magnified images of the same breast were compared. (Only three of the units were included since the Kramex had no grid or small focus.) The images from each unit were displayed in a single column with the contact view at the top and the magnified view at the bottom. Each column was labeled with the name of the unit.

Again the physicians were asked for their opinions. Most agreed that the grid images had more contrast than the nongrid images, but there was no strong preference for one unit over another.

Most felt that the 1.5X magnification provided as much diagnostic information as the 1.75X and 2X views and they expressed concern about using the higher doses required for the larger images.

Conclusions

For contact mammograms it appears that image quality and patient dose bear little relationship to the cost of the mammographic units tested. This suggests that for contact mammography, which makes up the bulk of clinical work, items other than dose and image quality should be considered when selecting a new unit, e. g., ease of positioning patients, availability of replacement parts and repair service, X-ray tube life, stability of automatic exposure system, degree of automatic density compensation, type and adequacy of operator shielding, range of programmed exposure factors, and tube loading limitations.

On the other hand, the higher priced units may incorporate features not available in the lower priced equipment such as a grid and/or a dual focus tube. A grid is clearly useful so the extra cost for this feature is well justified. Grids can now be obtained for use with the less expensive units.

The need for a small focal spot with its increased cost is more debatable. While some experts feel there is a definite advantage to magnification, in most clinical practices magnified views are used in only a small fraction of cases. There are other methods for obtaining good enlarged images at less cost and without subjecting the patient to extra radiation dose. These include the use of: (1) a hand magnifier or (2) a stereo zoom optical microscope equipped with an adjustable high-intensity light source (Galkin et al. 1983).

Acknowledgments. We would like to thank Drs. E. B. Go, W. Thorwarth, L. Woodruff, and the Elscint Corp. for making their mammographic units available.

We also appreciate the assistance provided by Joe Di Stefano, Newton Ganther, Thomas Keller, Patricia Masters, Lewin Mitchell, George Pulos, Randall Selah, Gale Sheldon, Gerald Stussman, Carl Thomsen, Virginia Wentz, and Dr. N. Yanaki.

References

Galkin B, Feig S, Frasca P et al. (1983) Photomicrographs of breast calcifications: correlation with histopathologic diagnosis. RadioGraphics 3: 3 450–477
Galkin B, Feig S, Frasca P et al. (1984) Imaging capabilities and dose considerations of different mammographic units (Abs.) Radiology 153: 365
Stanton L, Villafana T, Day J et al. (1984) Dosage evaluation in mammography. Radiology 150: 577–584

Computed Tomography Scanning, Transillumination, and Magnetic Resonance Imaging of the Breast

E. A. Sickles

Department of Radiology, Breast Imaging Section, University of California School of Medicine, San Francisco, CA 94143, USA

Each of the three breast imaging procedures discussed in this paper already has or may eventually have the ability to provide clinically useful information that complements the detailed anatomic information currently available from X-ray mammography. None of these procedures is expected to replace mammography as the first-line imaging technique for the detection and diagnosis of benign and malignant breast lesions. Computed tomographic (CT) scanning utilizes ionizing radiation to produce high-contrast images in a cross-sectional display. A few special indications for the procedure already have been established, applying to a very small percentage of mammography patients. However, it is unlikely that the technique will find much more widespread use in the future. Transillumination and magnetic resonance imaging do not use ionizing radiation, and are as yet unproved methods for breast cancer diagnosis.

Breast CT Scanning

Computed tomography scanning has gained acceptance as a diagnostic imaging procedure primarily by virtue of its ability to portray density differences much smaller than those demonstrable by conventional plain-film X-ray techniques. Unfortunately, this does not work in examining the breast because there is considerable overlap in the CT numbers of many breast cancers, several benign breast lesions, and dense collections of normal fibroglandular breast tissue (Gisvold et al. 1977; Chang et al. 1977). Only by imaging the breasts twice, both before and after intravenous iodide administration, can CT scanning produce levels of diagnostic accuracy comparable with X-ray mammography. It has been shown that the great majority of breast cancers demonstrate at least a 5% increase in CT number following iodide administration, whereas most benign lesions do not (Chang et al. 1980). Thus, contrast enhancement represents the principal CT criterion for the differentiation of benign from malignant lesions. Absolute values of CT numbers as well as shape and size of high-density areas are of lesser importance. Cancers presenting mammographically as tiny clustered calcifications without an associated mass are not identified on pre-iodide scans because CT scanning cannot resolve such small structures; however, many of these cancers are imaged on post-iodide scans as minute area(s) of substantial contrast enhancement.

Two prototype units of a dedicated breast CT scanner were evaluated in the late 1970s. Clinical trials with one unit demonstrated slightly increased cancer detection for CT scanning over mammography (Chang et al. 1980), whereas the other showed no difference (Gisvold et al. 1979). However, it was clear that CT scanning was inappropriate as a primary diagnostic test for breast cancer, because of the extremely high cost of examination, the need for intravenous iodide administration, and the relatively large radiation doses involved. As a result, the prototype scanners were dismantled and are no longer available.

Although breast CT imaging with a whole-body scanner can produce results similar to those obtained with the dedicated breast units (Chang et al. 1982), this technique is rarely if ever used for purposes of cancer detection and diagnosis. Not only does whole-body scanning of the breasts carry the disadvantages of very high cost and need for iodide administration, but it also imparts a substantially greater radiation dose and requires an unacceptably long time for image interpretation (Sickles 1983).

Despite the lack of general clinical utility for breast CT scanning, there are several specific, narrowly defined situations in which the examination can prove helpful. By virtue of its cross-sectional image display, it can be used to achieve prebiopsy localization of the rare nonpalpable mammographic lesion that is so close to the chest wall as to be visible on only one mammographic projection (Kopans and Meyer 1982; Dixon 1983). Because it readily indicates chest wall thickness and also may demonstrate the position of the internal mammary lymph node chains, its use has been advocated in treatment planning for women who receive radiotherapy for primary breast cancer (Munzenrider et al. 1979). Most importantly, CT scanning has utility among patients with known breast cancer in evaluating for subclinical metastasis to regional lymph nodes and to deeper structures by contiguous tumor spread. Indeed, thoracic CT imaging can provide the only indication of adenopathy in the internal mammary, axillary, mediastinal, and hilar nodes, of sternal or rib erosion, and of tumor invasion into the retromammary space and pectoral muscles. Detection of unsuspected metastasis in any of these locations can be of great value either in preoperative tumor staging (Muller and van Waes 1981) or in altering radiation treatment portals among patients with recurrent tumor (Meyer and Munzenrider 1981; Lindfors et al. 1985).

It is doubtful that breast CT scanning ever will achieve widespread clinical use. Much more likely its application will be limited to the specific clinical situations outlined above. There is, however, considerable promise in further elucidating the physiological processes that cause malignant (and perhaps also premalignant) breast tissue to have an increased affinity for iodide (Chang et al. 1978; 1980). The potential imaging consequences of such investigations range from the development of improved strategies for breast CT scanning to the synthesis of successful paramagnetic contrast agents for magnetic resonance imaging of the breast (see below).

Transillumination

Breast transillumination is accomplished by passing a beam of visible light through the breast and observing or recording the exiting signal. There have been several successive improvements in the design of transillumination equipment over the past 57 years since the pioneer investigations of Cutler (1929). Current techniques selectively utilize the far-red and near-infrared region of the spectrum because these longer-wavelength photons penetrate more readily through breast tissue. In addition, it is thought that there may be preferential light absorption by breast cancer in this portion of the spectrum, so that areas of malignancy absorb more (and therefore transmit less) light than do benign tissues (Sickles 1983).

Two major breast transillumination techniques are currently in use. One records images on infrared-sensitive photographic color film (Ohlsson et al. 1980; Isard 1981). The advantage of this approach is its relatively low cost, but the film must be developed by a chemical process that is provided by only a few commercial photographic laboratories, resulting in delays of up to a week or more before images are available for interpretation. With the other technique images are recorded by a television camera especially sensitive to far-red and near-infrared wavelengths (Watmough 1982; Bartrum and Crow 1984). This results in real-time viewing using a standard television monitor, with hard-copy recording of images on videotape or by taking Polaroid photographs off the television screen. Post-acquisition signal processing has been incorporated into some equipment, providing images that indicate the relative amounts of infrared-to-red transmission (in false color) in addition to total light transmission (Merritt et al. 1984). Such sophisticated devices are quite expensive, approaching the cost of state-of-the-art mammography equipment.

Using either film or television technique, cysts are identified as areas of increased light transmission, whereas solid tumors characteristically show as focal dark shadows because they demonstrate increased light absorption. Less specific transillumination signs of abnormality include changes in subcutaneous blood vessels, vague areas of asymmetrical light absorption, and retraction or thickening of the skin.

The primary theoretical limitation to transillumination techniques is that only a very small portion of the incident light, if any, is transmitted in a straight path through the breast. Thus, the great majority of photons are scattered extensively, thereby producing low-resolution images (Kopans 1984). The fact that current equipment uses large-area light sources and short imaging distances further degrades the transillumination image.

These theoretical principles are borne out by clinical experience, which indicates that only very superficially located structures are imaged clearly. Indeed, firm compression of the breast in a variety of different positions is required in order to visualize many lesions, especially small ones, by bringing them as close as possible to the skin surface through which the light beam exits (Bartrum and Crow 1984; Marshall et al. 1984; Sickles 1984). This makes the success of transillumination highly dependent on the skill of the operator, particularly if examination is done using a television-based system, in which real-time viewing of clinical images permits immediate adjustments in positioning and technical factors to optimize image quality. However, despite careful attention to these parameters, several pilot clinical studies using transillumination devices of different degrees of sophistication have consistently shown an inability to detect very small and deep-seated cancers (Bartrum and Crow 1984; Sickles 1984; Geslien et al. 1985; Drexler et al. 1985). These are the tumors that are most important to detect since they tend to be nonpalpable, just those lesions that are readily identified by mammography.

It is clear that current transillumination techniques have no role in screening for occult breast cancer, nor should any of them be used as an alternative to mammography in the evaluation of symptomatic patients. Several authors suggest clinical utility for transillumination in specific circumstances when mammography results in questionable or equivocal findings (Merritt et al. 1984; Geslien et al. 1985; Drexler et al. 1985). However, these recommendations are supported only by anecdotal experience; there has been no conclusive demonstration that transillumination can serve as an adjunct to mammography and physical examination in the evaluation of either symptomatic or asymptomatic patients. A large-scale multi-institution phase II clinical trial is underway to determine whether there is a role for breast transillumination, but results from this study will not be available for several years. At the present time, the examination has no established clinical indications and therefore remains an investigational tool.

It is unlikely that current transillumination devices will gain widespread clinical acceptance, because they do not overcome the limiting problem of light scattering. However, several scatter-reduction methods offer promise and should be further investigated. One such method would minimize scattering simply by reducing the volume of breast tissue illuminated. This involves the use of a narrow-beam light source, in effect examining only a small portion of the breast at a time. Such an approach will have the potential for clinical applicability only if equipment can be developed to scan rapidly and reliably over the entire breast to form composite whole-breast images. Another technique to reduce light scattering utilizes as a source beam the coherent light of an ultra-fast (picosecond) pulsed laser. Because scattered light travels a longer path than unscattered light, it takes a slightly longer time to traverse the breast. By gating image collection to the very brief picosecond pulses of incident light, it may be possible to record only the earliest component of each pulse to exit the breast, that which is least scattered.

In addition to developing scatter-reduction techniques, the basic physical properties of light absorption in the breast also should be investigated. By determining and comparing absorption spectra for the full range of cancers, benign lesions, and normal structures, it may be possible to define a range of wavelengths or series of wavelength ranges with which to image in order to maximally discriminate cancers from surrounding benign tissues.

Magnetic Resonance Imaging

In vivo magnetic resonance imaging (MRI) of the breasts has been possible only for the past 4 years, and current experience is far too incomplete to indicate whether it will play a significant role in the diagnosis of benign and malignant breast disease. Initial investigations were done using whole-body imaging coils (Ross et al. 1982; El Yousef et al. 1983; Sickles et al. 1983; El Yousef et al. 1984), with limited success. More recently, the development of high-resolution surface coils has resulted in superior breast images, capable of demonstrating smaller lesions and finer structural detail (El Yousef et al. 1984; El Yousef and Duchesneau 1984; Stelling et al. 1985; Wolfman et al. 1985; El Yousef et al. 1985; Alcorn et al. 1985; Dash et al. 1986). Indeed, the considerable degree of improvement in image quality with surface coils strongly suggests that all future breast MRI will be done using such high-resolution techniques.

Although limited in scope, current clinical experience with breast MRI already indicates many of its strengths and weaknesses. Fatty and fibroglandular regions of the breast are clearly distinguished, and areas of dense fibroglandular tissue are imaged with a greater range of contrast than either mammography or CT scanning. Large and some small breast lesions also are readily portrayed, especially if surrounded by substantial amounts of fatty tissue, with benign masses characteristically showing smooth, round, sharply defined margins and cancers demonstrating irregular and ill-defined borders (El Yousef et al. 1984). However, even when using surface coils, the spatial resolution of MRI is far inferior to mammography, so that the tiny clustered calcifications of intraductal carcinoma and the fine spiculations of invasive breast cancer are not imaged. There has also been difficulty in identifying some masses adjacent to dense areas of fibroglandular tissue. Not only for these reasons, but especially because of the very high cost of examination, it is exceedingly unlikely that MRI will be used for breast cancer screening (Kopans 1984; Dash et al. 1986).

Rather, breast MRI offers considerable promise in breast disease diagnosis, as a complement to mammography and physical examination. Even though MRI appears to be both sensitive and specific in the diagnosis of simple benign cysts (Stelling et al. 1985; El

Yousef et al. 1985; Alcorn et al. 1985; Dash et al. 1986), this is probably not a role for which it will find widespread clinical use, because of its high cost relative to the established techniques of aspiration and sonography. However, currently there is no test short of open biopsy that reliably excludes the diagnosis of malignancy for solid masses. If MRI can provide this ability, even if only for several specific benign lesions, it will prove to be a valuable adjunct to the standard diagnostic evaluation.

Current clinical investigations of breast MRI are beginning to address this important issue. Unfortunately, little progress has been achieved to date. Attempts to distinguish benign from malignant solid masses solely on the basis of their morphological features have not met with great success (El Yousef et al. 1985; Alcorn et al. 1985; Heywang et al. 1985). Indeed, MRI is less accurate than mammography in this regard, a situation that is hardly surprising since mammography has the greater spatial resolution. Parallel efforts also have failed to differentiate benign from malignant disease simply on the basis of variations in lesion intensity using different MR radiofrequency pulse sequences (Alcorn et al. 1985). Apparently there is too much overlap between the T_1 and T_2 values of benign and malignant lesions for these data to be used to direct clinical decisions. However, although it seems that neither morphological criteria nor quantitative MR parameters are sufficiently reliable independent diagnostic discriminators, preliminary evidence suggests that a synthesis of the information provided by both approaches may produce acceptable clinical results (El Yousef et al. 1985; Heywang et al. 1985).

It must be remembered that compared with the relatively mature modalities of CT scanning and transillumination, that breast MRI truly is in its infancy and that there are many potentially fruitful lines of investigation that have not yet begun to be explored. These include the use of paramagnetic contrast agents (perhaps coupled to molecules with similar affinity for carcinoma as intravenously administered iodide), the imaging of nuclei other than hydrogen, and MR spectroscopy. It will be many years before the diagnostic potential of breast MRI is fully evaluated. Currently the technique has no established clinical indications.

References

Alcorn FS, Turner DA, Clark JW et al. (1985) Magnetic resonance imaging in the study of the breast. RadioGraphics 5: 631–652

Bartrum RJ Jr, Crow HC (1984) Transillumination lightscanning to diagnose breast cancer: a feasibility study. Am J Roentgenol 142: 409–414

Chang CHJ, Sibala JL, Gallagher JH et al. (1977) Computed tomography of the breast: a preliminary report. Radiology 124: 827–829

Chang CHJ, Sibala JL, Lin F et al. (1978) Preoperative diagnosis of potentially precancerous breast lesions by computed tomography breast scanner: preliminary study. Radiology 129: 209–210

Chang CHJ, Sibala JL, Fritz SL et al. (1979) Specific value of computed tomographic breast scanner (CT/M) in diagnosis of breast diseases. Radiology 132: 647–652

Chang CHJ, Sibala JL, Fritz SL et al. (1980) Computed tomography in detection and diagnosis of breast cancer. Cancer 46: 939–946

Chang CHJ, Nesbit DE, Fisher DR et al. (1982) Computed tomographic mammography using a conventional body scanner. Am J Roentgenol 138: 553–558

Cutler M (1929) Transillumination as an aid in the diagnosis of breast lesions. Surg Gynecol Obstet 129: 721–729

Dash N, Lupetin AR, Daffner RH et al. (1986) Magnetic resonance imaging in the diagnosis of breast disease. Radiology 146: 119–125

Dixon GD (1983) Preoperative computed-tomographic localization of breast calcifications. Radiology 146: 836

Drexler B, Davis JL, Schofield G (1985) Diaphanography in the diagnosis of breast cancer. Radiology 157: 41–44

El Yousef SJ, Alfidi RJ, Duchesneau RH et al. (1983) Initial experience with nuclear magnetic resonance (NMR) imaging of the human breast. J Comput Assist Tomogr 7: 215–218

El Yousef SJ, Duchesneau RH, Alfidi RJ et al. (1984) Magnetic resonance imaging of the breast: work in progress. Radiology 150: 761–766

El Yousef SJ, Duchesneau RH (1984) Magnetic resonance imaging of the human breast: a phase I trial. Radiol Clin North Am 22: 859–868

El Yousef SJ, O'Connell DM, Duchesneau RH et al. (1985) Benign and malignant breast disease: magnetic resonance and radiofrequency pulse sequences. Am J Roentgenol 145: 1–8

Geslien GE, Fisher JR, DeLaney C (1985) Transillumination in breast cancer detection: screening failures and potential. Am J Roentgenol 144: 619–622

Gisvold JJ, Karsell PR, Reese DF et al. (1977) Clinical evaluation of computerized tomographic mammography. Mayo Clin Proc 52: 181–185

Gisvold JJ, Reese DF, Karsell PR (1979) Computed tomographic mammography (CTM). Am J Roentgenol 133: 1143–1149

Heywang SH, Fenzl G, Hahn D et al. (1985) MR imaging of the breast: histopathologic correlation. Radiology 157 (P): 323

Isard HJ (1981) Diaphanography: transillumination of the breast revisited. In: Schwartz GF, Marchant D (eds) Breast disease: diagnosis and treatment. Elsevier/North-Holland, New York, pp 67–70

Kopans DB, Meyer JE (1982) Computed tomography guided localization of clinically occult breast carcinoma – the "N" skin guide. Radiology 145: 211–212

Kopans DB (1984) "Early" breast cancer detection using techniques other than mammography. Am J Roentgenol 143: 465–468

Lindfors KK, Meyer JE, Busse PM et al. (1985) CT evaluation of local and regional breast cancer recurrence. Am J Roentgenol 145: 833–837

Marshall V, Williams DC, Smith KD (1984) Diaphanography as a means of detecting breast cancer. Radiology 150: 339–343

Merritt CRB, Sullivan MA, Segaloff A et al. (1984) Real-time transillumination light scanning of the breast. RadioGraphics 4: 989–1009

Meyer JE, Munzenrider JE (1981) Computed tomographic demonstration of internal mammary lymph-node metastasis in patients with locally recurrent breast carcinoma. Radiology 139: 661–663

Muller JWT, van Waes PFGM (1981) Selective mammography with a standard whole body CT scanner. Presented at annual meeting of Radiological Society of North America, Chicago

Munzenrider JE, Tchakarova I, Castro M et al. (1979) Computerized body tomography in breast cancer. I. Internal mammary nodes and radiation treatment planning. Cancer 43: 137–150

Ohlsson B, Gundersen J, Nilsson DM (1980) Diaphanography: a method for evaluation of the female breast. World J Surg 4: 701–705

Ross RJ, Thompson JS, Kim K et al. (1982) Nuclear magnetic resonance imaging and evaluation of human breast tissue: preliminary clinical trials. Radiology 143: 195–205

Sickles EA (1983) Breast CT scanning, heavy-ion mammography, NMR imaging, and diaphanography. In: Feig SA, McLelland R (eds) Breast carcinoma. Current diagnosis and treatment. Masson, New York, pp 233–250

Sickles EA, Davis PL, Crooks LE (1983) NMR characteristics of benign and malignant breast tissues: preliminary report. Radiology 149 (P): 92

Sickles EA (1984) Breast cancer detection with transillumination and mammography. Am J Roentgenol 142: 841–844

Stelling CB, Wand PC, Lieber A et al. (1985) Prototype coil for magnetic resonance imaging of the female breast: work in progress. Radiology 154: 457–462

Watmough DJ (1982) A light torch for the transillumination of female breast tissues. Brit J Radiol 55: 142–146

Wolfman NT, Moran R, Moran PR et al. (1985) Simultaneous MR imaging of both breasts using a dedicated receiver coil. Radiology 155: 241–243

Recent Trends in Screen-Film Mammography: Technical Factors and Radiation Dose*

A. G. Haus

Health Sciences Division, Eastman Kodak Company, Corporate Place, 343 State Street, Rochester, NY 14650, USA

Introduction

The trend in screen-film mammography is toward high-contrast, high-resolution images. In this article technical factors associated with X-ray equipment and/or the screen-film combination which affects radiographic contrast, blurring (unsharpness), and noise will be reviewed. Radiation dose will be discussed in terms of measurement, calculation, and theoretical risk.

Radiographic Contrast

Radiographic contrast refers to the magnitude of the optical density difference between the structure of interest and its surroundings. Radiographic contrast is influenced by two factors: subject contrast and film contrast.

Subject contrast is the ratio of the X-ray intensity transmitted through one part of the breast to the intensity transmitted through a more absorbing adjacent part. Subject contrast is especially important in mammography because of the subtle differences in the soft tissue density of normal and pathologic structures of the breast. Equally important is the detection of minute details such as microcalcifications and the marginal structural characteristics of soft-tissue masses. Some of the factors affecting subject contrast include: (a) absorption differences in the breast (thickness, density, defined here as mass per unit volume, and atomic number), (b) radiation quality (tube target material, kVp setting, and total filtration), and (c) scattered radiation. Scattered radiation can be reduced with good compression and with grids.

Radiation Quality

For screen-film mammography, overhead tungsten target tubes, as used for conventional screen-film radiography, should not be used because the resulting subject contrast is too low. Only the use of dedicated X-ray untis with either a molybdenum target tube and molybdenum filter or a specially designed tungsten target tube with a beryllium window is recommended. Selection and use of the appropriate tube target material, added beam fil-

---

* This article is adapted in part from monograph *Screen-Film Mammography Update: X-ray Units, Breast Compression Grids, Screen-Film Characteristics and Radiation Dose* by A. G. Haus, copyright by the Eastman Kodak Company (1984).

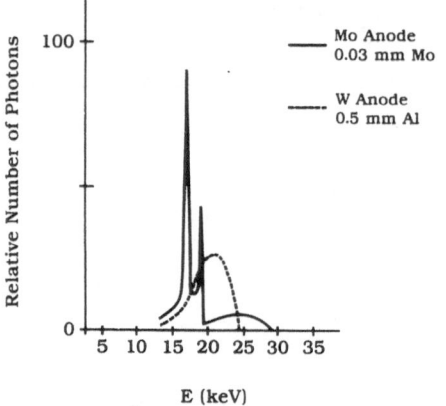

Fig. 1. Typical X-ray emission spectra (normalized to unit area) for screen-film mammography. This graph compares the spectra of a molybdenum *(Mo)* target (0.03-mm molybdenum filter, 28 kVp setting) and a tungsten *(W)* target (0.5-mm Al total filtration, 24 kVp setting). (Adapted from Haus 1983)

tration, and kVp setting are very important in order to achieve the high subject contrast which is necessary for screen-film mammography.

Figure 1 shows examples of emission X-ray spectra (normalized to unit area) when mammographic screen-film combinations are used (Haus et al. 1976; Fewell and Shuping 1978; Johnson and O'Fughludha 1980). These spectra illustrate typical beam quality characteristics. Dedicated molybdenum target X-ray units are widely used and settings of less than 28 kVp are generally recommended with these units. The use of low-energy photons, such as those produced by the 17.9 and 19.5 keV characteristic lines from the molybdenum target, provide high subject contrast for breasts of average thickness. When a 0.03-mm molybdenum filter is used, the spectrum is strongly suppressed at photon energies greater than 20 keV because of the k-shell absorption edge of molybdenum at that energy. Therefore, more radiation from the characteristic lines is used.

It is important to point out that the energy distribution of the image-forming photons transmitted through the breast strongly influences subject contrast (Haus et al. 1977; Fewell and Shuping 1978; Jennings et al. 1981). Clinically, for both the average-sized and predominantly fatty breast, a high percentage of low-energy photons are transmitted and utilized for recording the image when the molybdenum filter is used. Because of the greater filtering action of a thick dense breast, absorption differences among structures become smaller in the resulting "harder" X-ray beam. Therefore, subject contrast is not as high as with average-sized and fatty breasts.

If tungsten target tubes are used for screen-film mammography, only those specifically designed and dedicated for this application with beryllium windows and minimal aluminum filtration can be recommended. When the tungsten target tube is used, even at low-kVp settings, more high-energy photons are generally used in forming the image than for a molybdenum target tube. Therefore, it is most important to use low-kVp settings, preferably between 22 and 26 kVp. Although the breat-surface exposure may be low, subject contrast also can be expected to be low because the beam will have a higher average energy than the molybdenum target tube. When conventional overhead tungsten target tubes are used, excessive filtration and high-kVp settings account for most poor-quality screen-film mammograms, according to the Breast Exposure Nationwide Trends (BENT) study (Jans et al. 1979).

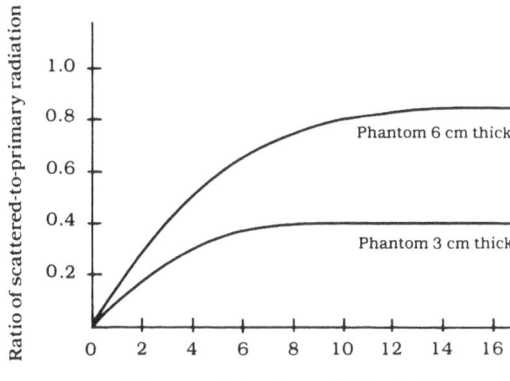

Fig. 2. Graph demonstrating dependence of the ratio of scattered-to-primary radiation on the diameter of the radiation field. *Curves illustrate values for 3 and 6 cm thicknesses of* a plastic breast phantom at 32 kVp. (Barnes et al. 1978)

Compression of the Breast

Good compression of the breast is a very important factor in reducing scattered radiation in screen-film mammography. Scattered radiation significantly reduces subject contrast in mammography especially for thick, dense breasts (Barnes 1979; Barnes and Brezovich 1978; Yester et al. 1981). Figure 2 shows the ratio of scattered-to-primary radiation for breast phantoms 6 cm and 3 cm thick as used in screen-film mammography (Barnes 1979). For the 6-cm-thick phantom and a 10-cm-diameter image field, intensity of scattered radiation reaching the image receptor is about 80% as great as the intensity of the primary radiation. Scattered radiation can be reduced by good compression. For example, if a 6-cm-thick breast (10-cm-diameter field) can be reduced to 3 cm (the diameter of the field is increased to approximately 14 cm), intensity of scattered radiation can be reduced to about 40% of the primary intensity for the same volume of irradiated tissue. By reducing the ratio of scattered-to-primary radiation, subject contrast is improved.

In addition to contributing to a reduction in scattered radiation, compression can provide several other technical improvements in image quality which can be achieved without compromising other image quality factors. These improvements include: (a) immobilization of the breast, which reduces blurring caused by motion, (b) location of structures in the breast closer to the image receptor, which reduces geometric blurring, (c) production of a more uniformly thick breast, which, in turn, results in more even penetration by X-irradiation and less difference in radiographic density in the area between the chest wall and the nipple, and (d) reduction of radiation dose. An added benefit is the spreading of breast tissue, which enables suspicious lesions to be more easily identified.

Grids for Mammography

The use of specially designed grids for mammography can further reduce scattered radiation and improve subject contrast, which is especially significant when imaging thick, dense breasts (Barnes and Brezovich 1978; Chan et al. 1983). Grids are now included with most of the new dedicated mammographic X-ray units. Some of these grids are of the reciprocating type, which blur the grid lines. Typical grid ratios are 5:1.

Focused stationary grids for mammography with ultra-high-strip density (80 lines/cm) have been evaluated recently (Chan et al. 1983) and are now commercially available (sup-

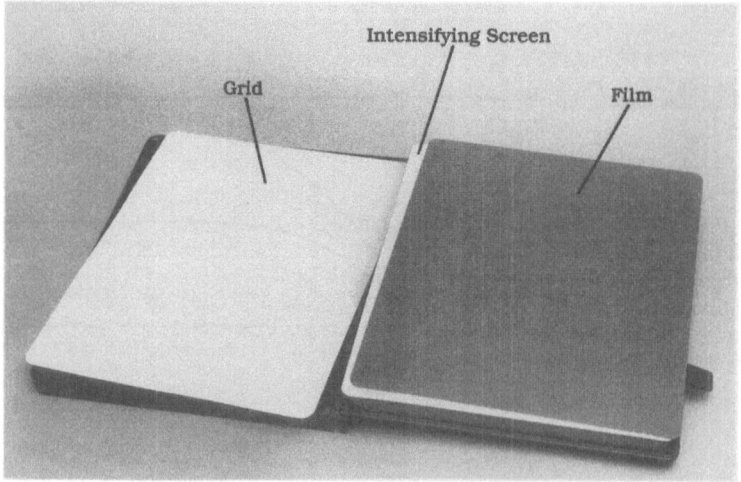

Fig. 3. Photograph of a stationary ultra-high strip density grid for mammography positioned within a Kodak Min-R cassette

plied by Liebel-Flarsheim, Cincinnati, Ohio). Typical stationary grid ratios are 3.5:1. These grids are about 1 mm thick and can fit inside cassettes designed for mammography (Fig. 3). The stationary grids can be used with any mammographic X-ray unit. They should be especially useful with mammographic units which cannot be retrofitted with a reciprocating grid. They are available in four sizes (18 × 24 cm, 24 × 30 cm, 8 × 10 incs., and 10 × 12 ins.) and for various focusing distances (37–47 cm, 44–58 cm, and 51–72 cm).

Grids designed for mammography require exposure increases ranging from approximately two to three times the exposures required for nongrid technics. This exposure increase can be accomplished by increasing the mAs setting. It may also be possible to offset the increased radiation exposure required when grids are used by using higher kilovoltage settings, increased beam filtration, or a recording system that provides higher speed, or with a combination of several factors.

Film Contrast, Speed

Film contrast characteristics determine how the X-ray intensity pattern will be related to the optical density in the mammogram. Film contrast is affected by film type, processing conditions (solutions, temperature, time, agitation), fog level (storage, safelight, light leaks), and the optical density (Fundamentals of Radiography 1980). Film contrast is defined in terms of the slope or steepness of the characteristic curve. The characteristic curves of three films recommended for mammography shown in Fig. 4 have sufficient contrast to cover the range of densities normally found in mammographic exposures. The steeper the curve, the higher the contrast. Note that of the three mammographic films shown, Kodak Ortho M Film has the highest contrast and also the highest speed.

Following the manufacturers' recommendations for film processing in terms of development time and temperature and processor maintenance are of critical importance in order to achieve and maintain appropriate film speed, film contrast, and film fog levels. Figure 5 illustrates the importance of film processing due to developer temperature

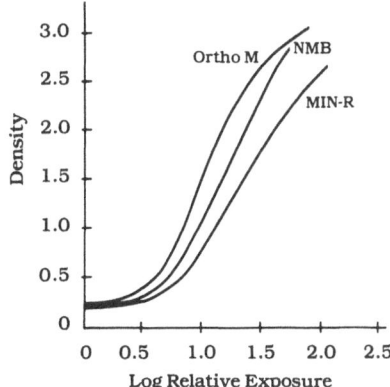

Fig. 4. Characteristic *curves* of Kodak Min-R, NMB, and Ortho M films exposed with a Kodak Min-R screen

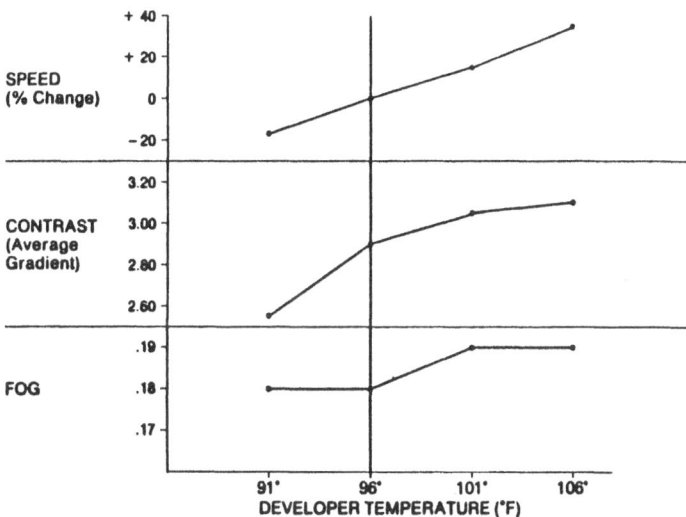

Fig. 5. Graph demonstrating percentage film speed change, film contrast (average gradient), and film fog plotted versus developer temperature. The *vertical line* indicates manufacturer's recommendations

differences on film speed, film contrast, and fog levels. Similar results could be expected if these variables were plotted versus development time. Note that when the developer temperature is lower than the manufacturer's recommendation, film speed is reduced. This loss in film speed may dictate an unnecessary increase in radiation dose in order to produce mammograms of proper optical density. Similiarly, film contrast is reduced when developer temperature is lowered. Conversely, if the developer temperature is higher than the manufacturer's recommendation, film speed is increased. This increase in film speed may permit a reduction in radiation dose. Film contrast may also be increased. Quantum mottle and therefore radiographic noise can be expected to increase due to increased film speed and higher film contrast. Film fog may increase with increased developer temperature. Developer stability may also be affected when developer temperatures higher than recommended are used.

Table 1. Example of exposure time increase adjustment due to the use of grid and reciprocity law failure effect

Present technic	1.0 s
Exposure time increase, grid or magnification	2.5X
Exposure increase due to reciprocity law failure (1→2.5 s)	15%
New technic, grid or magnification	2.9 s

Another factor relating to film speed is the effect of reciprocity law failure. Reciprocity law failure can be very important due to the trends in screen-film mammography of using long exposure times due to (1) use of grids, (2) use of small focal spots for conventional and magnification techniques (low-mA settings), and (3) use of a low-powered X-ray units with limited mA output settings. The definition given for Exposure ($E = I \times T$) states that the response of the film to radiation of a given quality will be unchanged if the product of intensity and time remains the same. It is implied that this relationship remains constant, regardless of whether long or short exposure times are used, provided that time changes are compensated for by a proportional change in intensity. This relationship, also known as the reciprocity law, does apply to direct exposures; however, for exposure to light, the law fails (Fundamentals of Radiography 1980). In mammography, reciprocity law failure may affect film density when long exposure times (approximately 1.0 s or longer) are used (Haus et al. 1979; Fundamentals of Radiography 1980). When reciprocity law failure effects occur, additional exposure may be required in order to provide the proper optical density on the mammogram. An example of technique adjustment due to the use of grid and reciprocity law failure effect is shown in Table 1.

Radiographic Blurring (Unsharpness)

Radiographic blurring refers to the lateral spreading of the image of a structural boundary; that is, to the distance over which the optical density change between the structure of interest and its surroundings takes place. Radiographic blurring results from three causes: motion, geometric, and screen-film blurring.

Motion Blurring

Motion blurring is caused by movement of the breast during exposure. It can be minimized by using a short exposure time and by firmly compressing the breast.

Geometric Blurring

Geometric blurring is affected by the size, shape, and intensity distribution of the X-ray tube focal spot in combination with focal spot-to-object and object-to-image receptor distances (Haus 1977). To minimize geometric blurring, the focal spot size and object-to-im-

Table 2. Nominal and measured equivalent focal spot sizes and focal spot-to-breast surface distances for several mammographic X-ray units

X-ray unit	Focal spot size (mm)		Focal spot-to-breast surface distance (cm)
	Nominal	Measured	
A	0.6	0.75 × 1.0	28
B	0.6	0.75 × 1.0	60
C	0.6	0.90 × 1.3	50
D	0.4	0.5 × 0.6	50
E	0.6	0.65 × 0.7	45
F	1.0	1.44 × 1.45	59
	2.0	2.50 × 2.90	59
G	0.45	0.70 × 0.85	44
	0.09	0.12 × 0.14	21

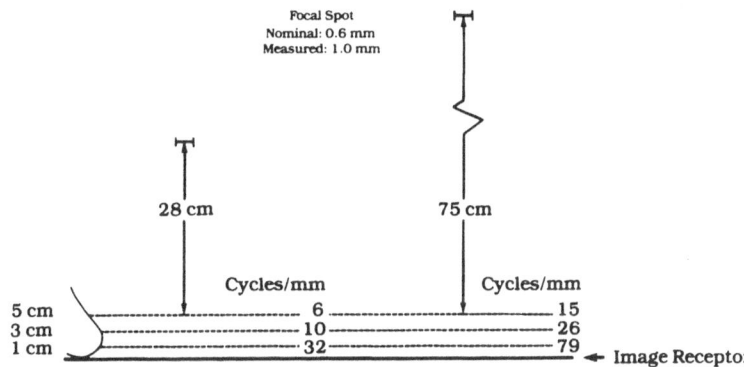

Fig. 6. Two equipment configurations for mammographic technics. Diagram compares situations where geometric blurring is a limiting factor *(left)* and has been reduced by increasing focal spot-to-object distance *(right)*. The limits of geometric resolution corresponding to object-to-image receptor distances of 5, 3, and 1 cm are shown. (Adapted from Haus 1984)

age receptor distance should be kept as small as possible, whereas focal spot-to-object distance should be maximized. Focal spot sizes and shapes for dedicated and conventional X-ray units used for mammography vary considerably as illustrated in Table 2 (Haus et al. 1978). Likewise, their focal spot-to-breast surface distance (cone lengths) vary considerably (Haus 1983). Table 2 shows the nominal focal-spot size provided by the manufacturer, the measured equivalent size determined with a star resolution pattern, and the focal spot-to-breast surface distance for two mammographic units. Focal spot size can be determined with a star resolution test object or pinhole camera (Braun 1978; Roeck and Milne 1978; Arnold et al. 1973).

Figure 6 illustrates the geometric configuration for a typical mammographic technic where geometric blurring is a limiting factor. The limit of geometric resolution corresponding to various planes in the breast can be calculated using the focal spot size, the distance from the focal spot size, the distance from the focal spot to the receptor, and the distance from the object to receptor (Haus et al. 1978; Haus et al. 1981). The limit of geometric resolution corresponding to object-to-image receptor distances of 1, 3, and 5 cm is 32, 10, and 6 cycles/mm, respectively.

Estimates of the recording system resolution can be obtained from MTF data or from bar-pattern resolution test objects. Most mammographic screen-film combinations have resolutions of about 15 cycles/mm (using the 4% MTF level as the criterion (Rossman 1964)). In this example, therefore, in order to make the recording system the limiting factor, the geometric resolution at an object-to-image receptor distance of 5 cm should exceed 15 cycles/mm.

According to the graph in Fig. 7, the focal spot-to-breast surface distance should be increased to approximately 75 cm as illustrated in Fig. 5 (Haus et al. 1978). Of course, this increase in distance must be compensated for by an increase in mAs and/or the use of a faster receptor. Figure 8 illustrates the resolution obtainable with a small focal spot, which is necessary to minimize the geometric blurring in magnification mammography that otherwise results from this technic (Haus et al. 1979).

uring the past few years, several studies (Haus 1977; Haus et al. 1978; Braun 1978) have indicated that the effect of geometric blurring is a significant limiting factor in ob-

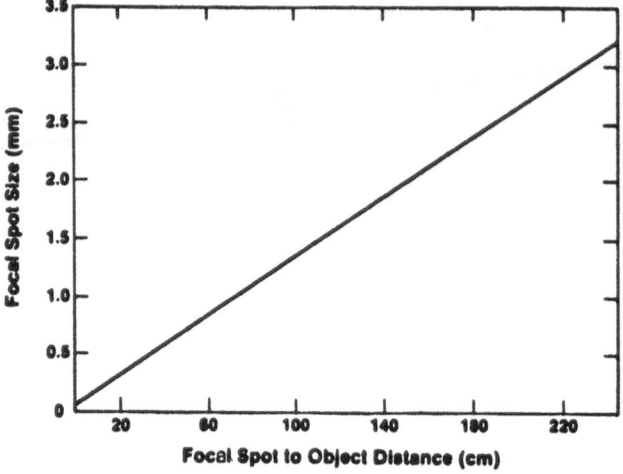

Fig. 7. Graph of equivalent focal spot size versus focal spot-to-object distance for a 5-cm object-to-recording system distance to achieve 15 cycles/mm of resolution

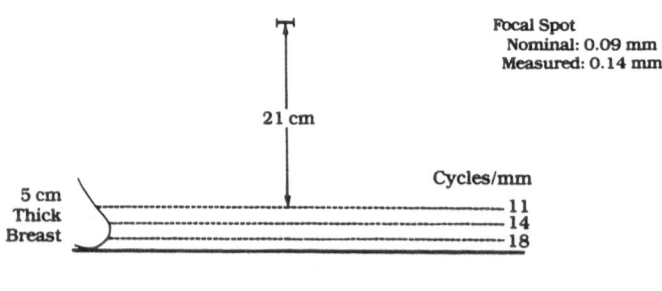

Fig. 8. Equipment configuration for a magnification technic (1.5 ×). For a 5-cm-thick breast, the geometric resolution limits corresponding to object-to-image receptor distances of 14, 12, and 10 cm are cited. (Adapted from Haus 1983)

taining maximum resolution of the breast image. This remains a limitation in some of the early dedicated mammographic units. While the current dedicated units are improved in this regard, some units could be improved to insure that the image receptor, and not geometric blurring, is the limiting factor in resolution.

Screen-Film Blurring

For screen-film mammography, light diffusion (spreading of the light emitted by the screen before it is recorded by the film) causes blurring. Factors involved include (a) screen phosphor thickness, (b) screen phosphor particle size, (c) light-absorbing dyes and pigments in the screen, and (d) screen-film contact (Fundamentals of Radiography 1980; Wayrynen 1979; Roth et al. 1979). The screen-film combination most commonly used in general medical radiography utilizes a double-coated film (with one emulsion on either side of the support) which is sandwiched between two intensifying screens (Fig. 9). Screen-film combinations for mammography utilize a single high-definition screen in contact with a single-emulsion film (Fig. 9). The single screen is used as a back screen for mammography. If the screen is used as a front screen, X-ray absorption is higher in the plane of the screen which is the furthest distance from the screen-emulsion contact surface. This causes greated light spread (blur) than when the X-ray absorption is highest near the screen-emulsion contact surface, as is the case when it is used as a back screen (Roth et al. 1979). Both parallax and crossover are eliminated in a single back-screen configuration, reducing blur and improving resolution. Cassettes designed for mammography have front panels which provide low X-ray absorption and provide intimate screen-film contact which also reduces blur (Fig. 3). Figure 10 shows modulation transfer function (MTF) curves for a mammographic screen-film combination (Kodak Min-R screen-Kodak Min-R film), and a double-emulsion, double-screen combination (Kodak Lanex regular screens-Kodak T-Mat G film). Note the significantly higher resolution for the mammographic combination. MTF curves for Kodak NMB or Kodak Orto M films exposed with Min-R screens are similar to the curve for the Min-R screen-Min-R film combination.

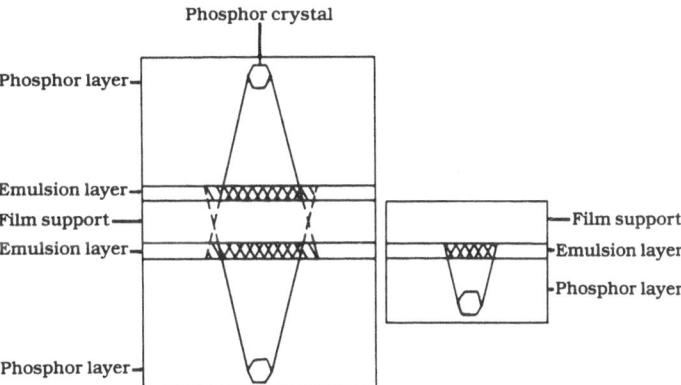

Fig. 9. Diagrams comparing physical configurations of two typical screen-film interfaces. A double-emulsion film (one emulsion on either side of the support) sandwiched between two intensifying screens *(left)* is used in general medical radiography. A single emulsion film in contact with a single back intensifying screen *(right)* produces excellent results in mammographic applications

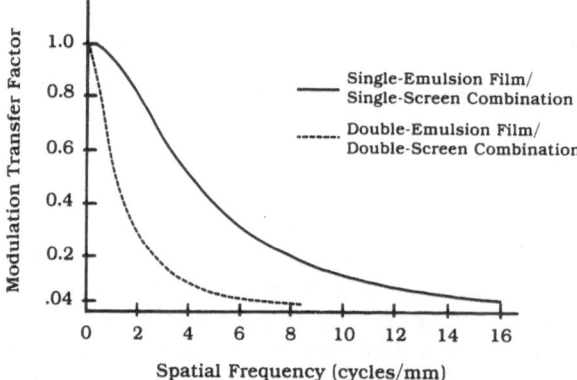

Fig. 10. Representative (MTF) *curves* for two typical screen-film combinations. *Curves* compare a double-emulsion film – double-screen combination (Kodak T-Mat G film – Kodak Lanex regular screens) used for general radiography with a single emulsion film – single screen combination (Kodak Min-R film – Min-R screen) designed for mammography

Radiographic Noise

Radiographic noise is unwanted fluctuation in optical density on the screen-film image (Fundamentals of Radiography 1980). Radiographic noise can be subdivided into two factors: (a) radiographic mottle and (b) artifacts.

Radiographic mottle is the optical density variation in a radiograph that has been given a uniform X-ray exposure. It consists of three components: (a) film graininess, (b) quantum mottle, and (c) structure mottle. Film graininess is the visual impression of the optical density variation due to the random distribution of the finite number of developed silver halide grains.

Quantum mottle is defined as the variation in optical density of a uniformly exposed radiograph that results from the random spatial distribution of the X-ray quanta absorbed in the image receptor. ("Uniformly exposed" means that the X-ray beam does not contain an object to be radiographed.) Quantum mottle is usually the principal contributor to the optical density fluctuation seen in a uniformly exposed radiograph.

Factors affecting quantum mottle include film speed and contrast, screen absorption and conversion efficiency, light diffusion, and radiation quality (Fundamentals of Radiography 1980). In mammography, quantum mottle may not be as limiting a factor relative to the graininess of direct exposure film as is commonly supposed because of the higher absorption by the screen of X-ray photons (approximately 80%) at low beam energies (Wayrynen 1979; Roth et al. 1979) illustrated in Table 3. A recent study (Barnes and Chakraborty 1982) suggests that because of the large photon flux and low energy levels used in screen-film mammography, the effect of quantum mottle in perception of radiographic detail may be less significant than that of film graininess. Consequently, for a given level of film graininess, it may be possible to reduce exposure without loss of information if film contrast is increased.

Table 3. Comparison of values for nominal exposure, fraction of X-ray beam absorbed, and effective exposure of a mammographic screen-film combination and a direct exposure film (data obtained at 30 kVp). (Adapted from Wayrynen 1979)

	Exposure (mAs)	Absorption (%)	Exposure × absorption[a]
Mammographic screen-film combination	25	80	20.0
Direct-exposure film	175	10	17.5

[a] Approximately proportional to number of X-ray quanta utilized.

Controlling Technical Factors

The technologist's role in the success of the screen-film mammographic examination is critical. Proper selection and control of technic factors including kVp setting, mAs, focal spot size, compression, geometry, and, most important, proper positioning are necessary. There is no diagnostic procedure where strict adherence to the prescribed technical factors is of more paramount importance. The quality of the mammogram is greatly dependent on the technologist's understanding of both technical factors and positioning and the ability to apply them carefully, correctly, and consistently.

Radiation Dose

In order to calculate the dose received during mammography, the exposure at the entrance surface of the breast for the technic used must be known. The most straightforward measurement that can be made is that of the exposure (roentgens) received at the entrance surface of the breast (at the bottom of the cone or the compression device employed) (Rothenberg et al. 1975).

The exposure measurement can be made with an ionization chamber or with thermoluminescent dosimeters (TLDs) (Rothenberg et al. 1975; Stanton et al. 1981). The ionization chamber method is considered to provide the more accurate results. Others (Rothenberg et al. 1975; Stanton et al. 1981; Lassen and Gorson 1981; Dubuque et al. 1977) have discussed in detail the equipment and the way it is used to measure the exposure at the entrance surface of the breast. The importance of proper calibration to assure accurate results with both methods, however, cannot be overemphasized. The tube output for typical exposure conditions should be measured periodically for quality assurance and whenever significant changes are made in the mammographic unit. The measurement should be made by a qualified medical physicist or an engineer.

Several years ago, it was common to use the exposure at the breast surface for comparison of various technics (for example, changes in kilovoltage and filtration of the beam) and image receptors. Recent studies have shown that exposure at the surface of the breast is not the most appropriate parameter for comparison of the radiation risk associated with various mammographic X-ray technics (Stanton et al. 1984, Hammerstein et al. 1979; Muntz 1979; NCRP Report 66 1980; Shrivastava 1981). *Absorbed dose* (in rads) received by the glandular tissue below the skin surface is more pertinent than surface exposure, because this is presumably the tissue at risk for the future development of cancer (Stanton et al. 1984, Hammerstein et al. 1979; Muntz 1979; NCRP Report 66 1980; Shrivastava 1981). Radiation dosage at a given depth depends on many factors: the ratio of glandular to fatty tissue (which decreases with the patient's age), the quality of the beam, the area of the breast irradiated (port sitze), and the exposure at the entrance surface of the breast. Several articles (Stanton et al. 1984, Hammerstein et al. 1979; Muntz 1979; NCRP Report 66 1980; Shrivastava 1981; Boag et al. 1976) containing depth doses for the low-energy X-ray beams used in mammography have been published.

Midbreast dose has been used in several studies to estimate the risk in mammography (Lester 1977; DHEW Publication (NIH) 77-1400 1977). In these studies, the surface exposure was derived without consideration of beam quality or breast composition. More recently, mean and integral doses have been considered better estimates of risk from mammography because they include the effects of beam quality and breast composition (Stanton et al. 1984; Hammerstein et al. 1979; Muntz 1979; NCRP Report 66 1980; Shrivastava 1981; Jones 1982).

Examples of typical entrance skin exposures and mean absorbed doses for a craniocaudal view when a Kodak MinR screen combined with a Kodak Min-R, NMB, or Ortho M film is used are shown in Table 4. For these measurements, radiographs of the Memorial BARTS breast phantom were made matching background optical densities at approximately 1.0. This phantom is 5 cm thick and consists of a preserved mastectomy specimen embedded in a block of tissue equivalent plastic (Malik et al. 1983; White et al. 1977; Miller and Masterson 1979). The base of the phantom is equivalent to 50% gland and 50% adipose. When exposed to an optical density of approximately 1.0 (over base + fog) the phantom requires an exposure similar to an average-sized breast. This phantom composition has been proposed as a standard when determining dose values for the purpose of comparing technics (Stanton et al. 1984). The entrance skin exposure in air was measured at the identical exposure conditions used for the phantom radiographs using an ionization chamber as discussed above. Mean doses to the mammary gland for a 5-cm-thick average breast per unit exposure in air are calculated using the appropriate conversion factor (Stanton et al. 1984; Hammerstein et al. 1979; Malik et al. 1983).

In 1976, Bailar assumed a midbreast dose of 2 rad to estimate the risk in mammography. This estimate was made without consideration of radiographic technic according to the receptors used. Results from the 27 screening centers of the joint American Cancer Society/National Cancer Institute Breast Cancer Detection Demonstration Project showed average midbreast doses for two-exposure examinations to be 0.08 rad for screen-film and 0.74 rad for xeroradiographic technics (Hammerstein et al. 1979; DHEW Publication

Table 4. Entrance skin exposures and mean absorbed dose comparisons of Kodak films used with Kodak Min-R Screen for mammography

Film	Entrance skin exposure (roentgens)	Mean absorbed dose (rad)
MIN-R	0.8	0.09
NMB	0.6	0.07
Ortho M	0.4	0.05

Mo target tube, 0.03-mm Mo filter, 28 kVp setting.

(NIH) 77-1400 1977). This translates into mid-breast doses of 1/25 (screen-film) and 1/3 (xeroradiography) of the doses used for the Bailar estimates of risk. As discussed previously, however, mean dose to the breast is considered to be a better indicator of risk.

A recent article by Feig discusses theoretical risk using low-dose mammography (Feig 1983). The following two paragraphs are quoted from this article.

Examination with current low dose technic (mean breast dose of 0.17 rad for a two-view study) would carry a theoretical risk of about one excess cancer case/year/2 million women examined. Assuming a 50 percent breast cancer mortality rate, the hypothetical risk would be one excess death/ 4 million women examined. This level of risk, one death/4 million women/year, is extremely small and can be equated with the following: 100 miles traveled by air, 15 miles traveled by car, smoking one-forth of one cigarette, one-third minute of mountain climbing, and 5 minutes of being a man aged 60 (Pochin 1978). Another means of appreciating the very small risk from mammography is by comparison with the natural breast cancer incidence. A risk of one excess breast cancer per 2 million women examined can be compared with the much larger magnitude of the natural breast cancer incidence: 800 cases/million women/year at age 40, 1800 cases/million women/year at age 50, and 2500 cases/million women/year at age 65 (Seidman 1980).

Conclusion

For screen-film mammography only dedicated X-ray equipment and screen-film combinations designed for mammography are recommended. The goal when producing a mammogram is to obtain as much diagnostic information as possible while at the same time minimizing radiation dose to the patient. This often necessitates compromises. By optimizing factors that affect image quality through the use of such means as appropriate beam quality, compression, good geometry, and consideration of grids, high-quality images can be obtained at low dose to the patient. For radiation dose values it is most important to determine the mean absorbed dose to the breast based on correct measurements and calculations. Once the mean glandular dose is determined, it can be used to estimate theoretical risk.

Acknowledgements. The author wishes to thank Ms. Pat Barnette for providing the helpful discussion on the section "Controlling Technical Factors." The author also gratefully acknowledges Mr. Douglas J. Crockett and Ms. Teresa J. Stich for their editorial contributions and Ms. Lynda Ingraham for typing the manuscript.

References

Arnold BA, Bjarngard BE, Klopping JC (1973) A modified pinhole camera method of investigation of X-ray tube focal spots. Phys Med Biol 18: 540–549

Barnes GT, Brezovich IA (1978) The intensity of scattered radiation in mammography. Radiography 126: 243–247

Barnes GT (1979) Characteristics of scatter. In: Logan WW, Muntz EP (eds) Reduced dose mammography. Masson, New York, pp 223–242

Barnes GT, Chakraborty DP (1982) Radiographic mottle and patient exposure in mammography. Radiology 145: 815–821

Boag JW, Stacey AJ, Davis R (1976) Radiation exposure to the patient in xeroradiography. Br J Radiol 49: 253–261

Braun M (1978) X-ray tube performance characteristics and their effect on radiologic image quality (recent and future trends in medical imaging). Proc Soc Photo-Opt Instrum Engineers 152: 94–103

Chan HP, Sepahdari S, Doi K (1983) Physical and clinical evaluation of ultra-high strip-density grids in mammography. Radiology (abstract) 149: 277 (Special Edition)

DHEW Publication (NIH) 77-1400 (1977) Final reports of national cancer institute ad hoc working groups on mammography screening for breast cancer and a summary report of their joint findings and recommendations. US Government Printing Office, Washington, DC

Dodd GD (1981) Radiation detection and diagnosis of breast cancer. Cancer 47: 1766-1769

Dubuque GL, Cacak RK, Hendee WR (1977) Backscatter factors in the mammographic energy range. Med Phys 4: 397-399

Feig SA (1983) Low-dose mammography: assessment of theoretical risk. In: Feig SA, McLelland R (eds) Breast carcinoma: current diagnosis and treatment. Masson, New York, pp 69-76

Fewell TR, Shuping RE (1978) A comparison of mammographic x-ray spectra. Radiology 128: 211-216

Fewell TR, Shuping RE (1978) HEW publication (FDA) 79-8071), (Handbook of mammographic x-ray spectra)

Fundamentals of Radiography (1980) Health Sciences Markets Division, Eastman Kodak Company, Rochester, Twelfth Edition

Hammerstein GR, Miller DW, White DR et al. (1979) Absorbed radiation dose in mammography. Radiology 130: 485-491

Haus AG, Metz CE, Chiles JT et al. (1976) The effect of x-ray spectra from molybdenum and tungsten target tubes on image quality in mammography. Radiology 118: 705-709

Haus AG, Metz CE, Doi K (1977) Determination of x-ray spectra incident on and transmitted through breast tissue. Radiology 124: 511-513

Haus AG (1977) The effect of geometric unsharpness in mammography and breast xeroradiography. In: Logan WW (ed) Breast carcinoma. The Radiologist's expanding role. Wiley, New York, pp 93-108

Haus AG, Cowart RW, Dodd GD et al. (1978) A method of evaluating and minimizing geometric unsharpness for mammographic x-ray units. Radiology 128: 775-778

Haus AG, Paulus DD, Dodd GD et al. (1979) Magnification mammography: evaluation of screen film and xeroradiographic techniques. Radiology 133: 223-226

Haus AG, Meyer J, Guebert DK (1981) Evaluation of the resolution limit for radiological procedures. In: Gray JE, Haus AG, Properzio WS, Mulvaney JA (eds) Application of optical instrumentation in medicine IX. Proc Soc Photo-Opt Instrum Engineers 273: 177-185

Haus AG (1983) Physical principles and radiation dose in mammography. In: Feig SA, McLelland R (eds) Breast carcinoma: current diagnosis and treatment. Masson, New York, pp 99-114

Jans RJ, Butler PF, McCrohan JL Jr (1979) The status of film-screen mammography. Results of the BENT Study. Radiology 132: 197-200

Jennings RJ, Eastgate RJ, Siedband MP (1981) Optimal x-ray spectra for screen-film mammography. Med Phys 8: 629-639

Johnson GA, O'Foghludha F (1980) Simulation of mammographic x-ray spectra. Med Phys 7: 189-195

Jones CH (1982) Methods of breast imaging. Phys Med Biol 27: 463-499

Lassen M, Gorson RO (1981) Patient dose in diagnostic radiology (refresher course handout at 67th Scientific Assembly and Annual Meeting of the Radiological Society of North America, Chicago)

Lester RG (1977) Risk versus benefit in mammography. Radiology 124: 1-6

Malik S, Masterson ME, Hunt M (1983) Effects of kVp variation and x-ray tube filtration on the mammographic examination application of optical instrumentation in medicine XI. Proc SPIE 419: 42-50

Miller DW, Masterson ME (1979) Mammography phantom development at the northeast center for radiological physics. In: Logan WW, Muntz EP (eds) Reduced dose mammography. Masson, New York, pp 307-308

Muntz EP (May/June) (1979) Relative carcinogenic effects of different mammography techniques. Med Phys 6: 205-210

NCRP Report 66 (1980) Mammography. National Council on Radiation Protection and Measurements, Washington, DC

Pochin EE (1978) Why be quantitative about radiation risk estimates? Lecture No 2: The Lauriston S. Taylor lecture series in radiation protection and measurements. National Council on Radiation Protection and Measurements

Roeck WW, Milne ENC (1978) A highly accurate focal spot camera – laboratory and field model. Radiology 127: 779–783

Rossman K (1964) Measurement of the modulation transfer function of radiographic systems containing fluorescent screens. Phys Med Biol 9 (4): 551–557

Roth B, Hamilton JF Jr, Bunch CP (1979) Fundamental aspects of mammographic photoreceptors: screens. In: Logan WW, Muntz EP (eds) Reduced dose mammography. Masson, New York, pp 529–536

Rothenberg LN, Kirch RLA, Snyder RE (1975) Patient exposures from film and xeroradiographic mammographic techniques. Radiology 117: 701–703

Shrivastava PN (1981) Radiation dose in mammography: an energy-balance approach. Radiology 140: 483–490

Siedband MP, Jennings RJ, Eastgate RJ (1977) X-ray beam filtration for mammography. In: Gray JE, Hendee WR (eds) Application of optical instrumentation in medicine VI. Proc Soc Photo-Opt Instrum Engineers 127: 204–207

Seidman H (1980) Statistical and epidemiological data on cancer of the breast. American Cancer Society, New York

Stanton L, Day JL, Bratteli SD et al. (1981) Comarison of ion chamber and TLD dosimetry in mammography. Med Phys 8: 792–798

Stanton L, Villafana T, Day JL et al. (1984) Dose evaluation in mammography. Radiology 150: 577–584

Wayrynen RE (1979) Fundamental aspects of mammographic receptors film process. In: Logan WW, Muntz EP (eds) Reduced dose mammography. Masson, New York, pp 521–528

White DR, Martin RJ, Darlison R (1977) Epoxy resin based tissue substitutes. Br J Radiol 50: 814–821

Yester MV, Barnes GT, King MA (1981) Experimental measurements of the scatter reduction obtained in mammography with a scanning multiple slit assembly. Med Phys 8: 158–162

Comparison of Mammographic Screen-Film Systems

E. A. Sickles

Department of Radiology, Breast Imaging Section, University of California School of Medicine, San Francisco, CA 94143, USA

In 1973 the DuPont Lo-dose screen-film system was introduced, to offer a lower-dose alternative to direct exposure film mammography and xeromammography (Ostrum et al. 1973; Weiss and Wayrynen 1976). When used with a molybdenum-anode dedicated mammography unit, vigorous breast compression, and proper breast positioning, the resulting images appeared to contain as much diagnostic information as those produced by the established mammographic techniques. As a result, the DuPont Lo-dose system gained acceptance by many mammographers.

Second-Generation Screen-Film Combinations

Three years later, primarily in response to the then raging controversy over the potential radiation hazards of mammography, several other even faster screens and films were developed, to allow for further dose reductions. With the existence of a variety of screen-film systems, having somewhat different imaging properties, came the need for comparative evaluations to determine whether the reduced dose of the newer systems was accompanied by clinically significant amounts of image degradation. Specifically sought was the screen-film combination that provided the highest level of diagnostic accuracy at the lowest radiation dose.

At the University of California in San Francicso we designed parallel laboratory and clinical studies to accomplish just this purpose. First we compared the imaging properties (resolution, contrast, noise) of four lower-dose recording systems to DuPont Lo-dose (Sickles et al. 1977). The second portion of the study evaluated the abilities of the various recording systems to portray the clinically relevant features of the mammographic image and also to assess overall accuracy of diagnostic interpretation (Sickles and Genant 1979).

We tested the five screen-film combinations listed in Table 1. Each was loaded into vacuum-sealed light-tight thin plastic envelopes to insure effective screen-film contact with minimum attenuation of the X-ray beam. All mammograms were taken by the same technologist, using the same molybdenum-anode X-ray unit, at the same source-image distance, using the same kVp and exposure time. Only the tube current (mA) was adjusted for each patient, to allow for differences in breast thickness and density. All films were developed in the same automatic processor.

We studied 100 consecutive mammography patients. After completion of conventional (DuPont Lo-dose) mammography, four additional craniocaudal projection mammograms were taken of the more symptomatic or otherwise more abnormal breast, using each of the lower-dose screen-film combinations. This provided five craniocaudal projection mammograms of each patient to use for clinical evaluation. All image interpretation

Table 1. Screen-film combinations tested[a]

Screen	Film	Combination
DuPont Lo-dose	DuPont Lo-dose	Lo-dose
DuPont Lo-dose-2	DuPont Lo-dose	Lo-dose-2
Kodak Min-R	Kodak Min-R	Min-R
Kodak Min-R	Kodak NMB[b]	Min-R/Nuc Med
3M Alpha 4	Kodak Min-R	Alpha-4/Min-R

[a] Only films made in the United States were tested. The manufacturers produce similar but not identical films in Europe, sometimes using the same brand names. Therefore, results from this study do not necessarily apply to European-made films, even ones carrying the same names.

[b] *NMB*, Nuclear Medicine B.

Table 2. Criteria for random-order evaluation

Physical parameters	Anatomical parameters
Resolution (detail)	Normal breast structures
– Optimal	– Optimally visualized
– Adequate	– Adequately visualized
– Poor, but diagnostic	– Poorly shown, but diagnostic
– Unacceptable	– Not visualized
Contrast	Breast mass(es)
– Optimal	– Optimally visualized
– Adequate	– Adequately visualized
– Poor, but diagnostic	– Poorly shown, but diagnostic
– Unacceptable	– Not visualized
Noise (mottle)	Breast microcalcifications
– No noise visible	– Optimally visualized
– Minimal noise	– Adequately visualized
– Poor, but diagnostic	– Poorly shown, but diagnostic
– Unacceptable	– Not visualized

was done in single-blind fashion, with two radiologists working indepedently, under standard viewing conditions including the use of a 2X magnifying lens. Criteria for evaluation are listed in Table 2. Initially, all 500 images were evaluated in random order. Then, maintaining the random order of screen-film combinations, the five films from each patient were grouped together for evaluation-by-rank, using the same parameters listed in Table 2 but according to criteria ranging from "best visualized" (rank 1) to "most poorly visualized" (rank 5). For the ranking of image quality, rank 1 represented the greatest resolution, most contrast, and least noise.

Radiation exposure (entrance skin dose) was measured for the first 40 study patients by thermoluminescent dosimetry (Table 3). These values then were used to calculate ab-

Table 3. Radiation dose per exposure (40 patients)

Screen-film combination	Entrance skin dose (R)	Mid-breast dose (rad)	Mean dose to glandular tissue (rad)
Lo-dose	1.26	0.09	0.15
Lo-dose-2	0.64	0.05	0.07
Min-R	0.57	0.04	0.07
Min-R/Nuc Med	0.52	0.04	0.06
Alpha-4/Min-R	0.37	0.03	0.04

sorbed dose to the glandular tissue of the breast. Each of the faster screen-film combinations demonstrated two to three times lower radiation dose than the original DuPont Lo-dose system.

Parallel laboratory studies of resolution, contrast, and noise were carried out for all the screen-film combinations tested. Resolution was evaluated qualitatively by radiographing a set of microwire meshes (ranging from 4 to 20 line pairs per millimeter) and quantitatively by measuring modulation transfer functions. Determinations of contrast were derived from transmission densitometry measurements made on radiographs taken with a Lucite step wedge having 2-mm increments of thickness. System noise was estimated qualitatively by radiographing 2- to 3-mm-diameter plastic bead test objects and quantitatively by deriving Wiener spectra. Results of all these laboratory studies closely paralleled those obtained clinically from the subjective single-blind evaluations of image quality described below in detail.

Results of the clinical evaluations of resolution, contrast, and noise are presented in Tables 4–6, respectively. For resolution, very similar findings were recorded for all the screen-film combinations except the Alpha-4/Min-R combination, which was judged poorer in 25% of the films in the random-order evaluation. The Min-R/Nuclear Medicine combination was found to have the highest contrast, with both the Lo-dose and Lo-dose-2 systems rated poorest in this regard. Results for noise were almost exactly opposite those for contrast, with the Lo-dose system top-rated and the Min-R/Nuclear Medicine combination found to be most noisy. It is important to note that in none of the evaluations were the resolution, contrast, or noise of any of the screen-film combinations judged to be unacceptably poor.

All of the screen-film combinations portrayed the skin, nipple, areola, and internal breast architecture with approximately equal clarity. Both random-order and rank evaluations of the visibility of these structures showed differences in ratings of less than 5%.

Masses were seen in 22 of the 100 patients, on all 5 films for each patient except one, in whom the mass was located so close to the chest wall that it simply was not included on one image. Results of the clinical evaluations for masses are shown in Table 7. There were only very small differences among the Lo-dose, Lo-dose-2, and Min-R systems, with slightly poorer ratings for the other two combinations.

Results of the analyses of microcalcifications are presented in Table 8. Three or more calcific particles were identified on all 5 films in 36 of the 100 study patients. There were minimal differences among the four top-rated screen-film combinations, with the Lo-dose system judged best among these, and the Alpha-4/Min-R combination rated slightly lower than the others.

By far the most important of all the clinical evaluations were those of diagnostic impression. These showed striking consistency, with no differences in final diagnosis among

Table 4. Single-blind evaluations of resolution (detail)

Screen-film combination	Random-order			Rank
	Optimal	Adequate	Poor, but diagnostic	Mean rank score[a]
Lo-dose	39	55	6	2.44
Lo-dose-2	37	56	7	2.89
Min-R	36	58	6	2.56
Min-R/Nuc Med	35	58	7	2.67
Alpha-4/Min-R	15	75	10	4.45

[a] Rank score closest to 1 represents greatest resolution.

Table 5. Single-blind evaluations of contrast

Screen-film combination	Random-order			Rank
	Optimal	Adequate	Poor, but diagnostic	Mean rank score[a]
Lo-dose	5	70	25	4.39
Lo-dose-2	5	77	18	4.17
Min-R	21	72	7	2.22
Min-R/Nuc Med	28	67	5	1.56
Alpha-4/Min-R	15	76	9	2.67

[a] Rank score closest to 1 represents highest contrast.

Table 6. Single-blind evaluations of noise (mottle)

Screen-film combination	Random-order			Rank
	Optimal	Adequate	Poor, but diagnostic	Mean rank score[a]
Lo-dose	6	92	2	1.06
Lo-dose-2	1	96	3	2.11
Min-R	1	84	15	3.06
Min-R/Nuc Med	0	38	62	4.83
Alpha-4/Min-R	0	62	38	3.94

[a] Rank score closest to 1 represents least noisy images.

Table 7. Single-blind evaluations of breast mass visualization

Screen-film combination	Random-order				Rank
	Optimal	Adequate	Poor, but diagnostic	Not seen	Mean rank score[a]
Lo-dose	2	14	5	79[b]	1.91
Lo-dose-2	3	14	5	78	1.89
Min-R	2	15	5	78	2.34
Min-R/Nuc Med	0	15	7	78	4.64
Alpha-4/Min-R	0	15	7	78	4.22

[a] Rank score closest to 1 represents breast mass best seen.
[b] In one patient, a breast mass located close to the chest wall was not included on the Lo-dose image.

Table 8. Single-blind evaluations of microcalcification visualization

Screen-film combination	Random-order				Rank
	Optimal	Adequate	Poor, but diagnostic	Not seen	Mean rank score[a]
Lo-dose	2	27	7	64	2.37
Lo-dose-2	0	28	8	64	3.06
Min-R	1	28	7	64	2.75
Min-R/Nuc Med	0	28	8	64	2.70
Alpha-4/Min-R	0	25	11	64	4.12

[a] Rank score closest to 1 represents microcalcifications best seen.

any of the tested screen-film combinations, except for the previously described case of a single film that failed to include the spiculated mass of a carcinoma close to the chest wall.

The major conclusion drawn from this study was that substantial dose reduction indeed can be obtained, without sacrifice in diagnostic accuracy, by using any of the four screen-film combinations tested. Although reduced dose was accompanied by slight degradation in image quality, this was of insufficient magnitude to affect mammographic interpretation. The study also provided objective clinical support for the large number of radiologists who then began to use lower-dose screen-film mammography techniques.

Third-Generation Screen-Film Systems

Several years later, a new generation of even faster mammography films was introduced, in part to provide further dose reduction but also permit imaging with shorter exposure time and/or longer source-image distance, both of which help to increase the sharpness of the mammographic image (Haus et al. 1975). Prominent in this group were Kodak Ortho M and DuPont MRF-31 films. Neither these films nor any of the others of this generation have been evaluated in a prospective controlled clinical trial similar to the one described above. However, there is fairly general consensus, based solely on individual observations, that high levels of diagnostic accuracy are maintained. Anecdotal experience indicates that the new generation of ultra-low-dose films achieve faster speed at the expense of additional system noise. They also exhibit increased contrast, even more so than the highest-contrast second-generation (Min-R/Nuclear Medicine) combination.

Future Developments

The same manufacturers that have provided us with second- and third-generation screen-film systems continue to develop even faster films. Most of these are never marketed, either because they produce or are perceived to produce significant amounts of degradation of the mammographic image. On the other hand, it is only a matter of time before the next generation of screen-film combinations becomes commercially available. When this occurs, eventual clinical acceptance should not be based simply on subjective assessments of image quality but rather on the ultimate clinical test: whether dose reduction is achieved without any sacrifice in diagnostic accuracy.

References

Haus AG, Doi K, Chiles JT et al. (1975) The effect of geometric and recording system unsharpness in mammography. Invest Radiol 10: 43–52

Ostrum BJ, Becker W, Isard HJ (1973) Low-dose mammography. Radiology 109: 323–326

Sickles EA, Genant HK, Doi K (1977) Comparison of laboratory and clinical evaluations of mammographic screen-film systems. In: Application of optical instrumentation in medicine VI. Society of Photo-Optical Instrumentation Engineers, Bellingham, pp 30–35

Sickles EA, Genant HK (1979) Controlled single-blind clinical evaluation of low-dose mammographic screen-film systems. Radiology 130: 347–351

Weiss JP, Wayrynen RE (1976) Imaging system for low-dose mammography. J Appl Photogr Engineer 2: 7–10

Screening for Breast Cancer: An Overview

L. Tabár

Mammographic Section, Department of Radiology, Falun Hospital, 79182 Falun, Sweden

The results from the randomized, controlled trial in New York in the 1960s (HIP study) provided strong evidence that the course of breast cancer can be altered by detecting and treating it at an early stage (Shapiro et al. 1971). Encouraged by these results, additional randomized controlled trials have been started in Sweden (Andersson et al. 1979; Bjurstam et al. 1985; Fagerberg et al. in press; Frisell et al. 1983; Tabár and Gad 1981), Canada (Miller et al. 1981) and Scotland (Roberts et al. 1984), in order to find out the effect of screening in different countries and the effect of different screening designs.

There has been a remarkable improvement in the examination methods of the breast, especially for mammography, during the 1970s and 1980s and assumptions were made regarding the benefits from these improvements. Mammography alone has convincingly demonstrated its ability to lower the diagnostic threshold substantially, i. e., to detect a large number of very small cancers. When using mammography as a screening method we can hope to prevent many breast cancers from developing to incurable stages.

However, there are various, well-known biases associated with screening (lead-time bias, length bias sampling, detection bias, etc.). This is why it is vital to perform population-based, randomized, controlled trials in order to avoid decision-making on the basis of assumed benefits. This is the best way to find out whether a significant number of advanced carcinomas can be eliminated as an effect of screening and whether significant reduction in mortality from breast cancer can be achieved. This gives importance to the ongoing randomized, controlled breast cancer screening trials.

There are substantial differences between different countries, concerning health care structure, attitude to population screening, and awareness of the disease. These necessitate finding the most suitable screening-organization strategy in order to examine as high a proportion of the female population as possible. Additionally, mortality from breast cancer differs from country to country (Cancer Statistics 1984). England and Wales lead the breast cancer mortality list. Sweden is 22nd on the list, mortality rate being substantially lower in Sweden than in England and Wales. Consequently, the potential to save lives may be greater in some countries. Thus, it is important to find out the magnitude of benefit in different countries when screening with mammography; similarly, it is important to find out the benefit of screening in bigger towns as compared with rural areas, within the same country. That is why the data collected by the ongoing randomized controlled trials are invaluable.

The combined Kopparberg-Östergötland trial in Sweden is the first randomized controlled trial which has demonstrated reduction in mortality from breast cancer after mass screening since the HIP study results reported. By adding the results of two nonrandomized Dutch studies (Colette et al. 1984; Verbeck et al. 1984) to the results of the HIP and Swedish randomized, controlled trials, one can conclude that "the key question concerning early detection has been answered clearly, unambiguously and beyond doubt. Early detection alters the natural history of the disease" (Moskowitz 1981). We have convincingly demonstrated that properly performed and interpreted mammography can detect breast cancer before it has grown to an incurable stage. The large-scale application of this capability can result in an substantial change of the breast cancer problem, such as:

1. Mortality caused by breast cancer can be lowered by more than 50% in the continually screened group as compared with the never-screened one.
2. Significantly better treatment can be offered to most breast cancer patients when the patient material originates from screening.
3. Additionally, screening is highly cost-effective for the society.

These achievements must arouse much attention both in public opinion and among professionals and can be considered an important landmark in medicine. Consequently, we have much work ahead of us and our tasks in the immediate future can be summarized as follows:

Information

1. *Proper information must be given to collegues in the medical profession.* Meetings, conferences, publications, etc. should spread the details of this very important achievement in medicine. All those who could be involved in future population screening programs, in some way or another – general practitioners, surgeons, radiologists, radiotherapists, pathologists, cytologists, oncologists, and many others – should be ready to handle all the specific problems screening brings about. Extensive knowledge has been accumulated in the screening centers and all of them are ready to share their experience with future screeners.
2. *Proper and sincere information must be given periodically to the public.*
   It is necessary to use the power of mass media for this purpose. What are the most important messages we want to get accross?
   a) *Every women* runs a risk of getting breast cancer and the overriding risk factor is *age.*
   b) Mammography cannot prevent breast cancer; consequently, *the examination must be repeated at regular intervals.*
   c) There is no diagnostic method in medicine with 100% accuracy. This is why *breast self-examination* plays an important role in detecting breast diseases in the interim period, between two consecutive screenings.
   Mammography is the most reliable method – in experienced hands – but the combination of properly performed and interpreted mammography as well as breast self-examination gives the best results available today.
Women have to feel themselves motivated to attend the screening examination and participate at regular intervals. How can we motivate them? (1) By letting them know that in case we discover a breast cancer at screening the risk of dying from that cancer is more than 50% less than it is among those women who never attend screening. (2) By informing the population about the alternative therapeutic methods which have a direct impact on the life quality of the breast cancer patient.

Standards

The other very important task is to ensure that the personnel entrusted with the responsibility of screening carry out this task to the *highest professional standard*. It is necessary to train enough radiographers and radiologists in the immediate future in order to open well-organized breast cancer screening centres where high-quality mammograms are taken and these are interpreted by well-trained radiologists.

Additionally, rapid and efficient diagnostic workup and treatment is needed to minimize psychological trauma. The psychological factor is especially important and certainly more emphasized in screening than in everyday practice because screening affects a broad spectrum of the healthy population.

Finally, it is important to realize that *screening with mammography can lead to reduction of health service costs*. It is clear that an advanced breast cancer case can be very expensive for the society; from the time of dissemination the expenses can be extremely high. A large proportion of these expenses are saved in the population invited to screening, as it is clearly demonstrated that properly performed screening results in a significantly decreased number of advanced breast cancers in the total study population as compared with the control group (Tabar et al. 1985a, b). However, screening itself drains the economic recources. The cost of screening outweighs the savings during the first 4 or 5 years, although, from year 5 and further on the expenses of screening are far less than the savings because of the significantly fewer advanced, costly cases. This is the experience in Kopparberg county, Sweden, where basic data concerning economy have been collected prospectively and the design of the study has given ideal opportunity for comparing the expenses and savings at any time-level in the total study and control populations.

References

Andersson I, Andren L, Hildell J, Linell F, Ljungquist U, Pettersson H (1979) Breast cancer screening with mammography. Diagn Radiol 132: 273–276

Bjurstam N, Cahlin E, Eriksson O, Hafström LO, Rudenstam CM, Säve-Söderberg J (1985) Two-view mammography. An efficient method for breast cancer screening. Report from the breast cancer screening project in Göteborg, Sweden. Abstracts. 3rd European conference on clinical oncology and cancer nursing, Stockholm

Cancer Statistics (1984) CA 34: 7–23

Colette HJA, Day NE, Rombach JJ, De Waard F (1984) Evaluation of screening for breast cancer in a non-randomised study (the DOM-project) by means of a case-control study. Lancet 1: 1124–1126

Fagerberg G, Baldetorp L, Gröntoft O, Lundström B, Månson JC, Nordensköld B (in press) The effects of repeated mammographic screening on breast cancer stage distribution. Results from a randomised study of 92,934 women in a Swedish county. Acta Radiol Oncol

Frisell J, Broberg A, Glas U, Hellström L (1983) A randomised mammographic screening trial in Stockholm: cancer incidence and tumor characteristics. Proceedings 3rd EORTC breast cancer working conference, Amsterdam

Lundgren B, Jacobsson S (1976) Single view mammography. A simple and efficient approach to breast cancer screening. Cancer 38: 1124–1129

Miller AB, Howe GR, Wall C (1981) The national study of breast cancer screening. Protocol for a Canadian randomised controlled trial of screening for breast cancer in women. Clin Invest Med 4: 277–285

Moskowitz M (1985) Do the results of the Swedish trial, the Dutch case control study and the Cincinatti breast cancer detection demonstration project tell us anything of importance about the natural history of breast cancer? In: Evaluation du risque de cancer mammaire Chimiothèrapie premiére? Proceedings of the international symposium of senology, Liege, Belgium, 7–9 Nov 1985

Roberts MM, Alexander FE, Andersson TJ, Forrest APM, Hepburn W, Huggins A, Kirkpatrick AE, Lamb J, Lutz W, Muir BB (1984) The Edinburgh randomised trial of screening for breast cancer: description of method. Br J Cancer 50: 77–84

Shapiro S, Strax P, Venet L (1971) Periodic breast cancer screening in reducing mortality from breast cancer. JAMA 215: 1777–1785

Tabár L, Gad A (1981) Screening for breast cancer: the Swedish trial. Radiology 138: 219–222

Tabár L, Fagerberg G, Gad A, Baldetorp L, Holmberg LH, Gröntoft O, Ljungquist U, Lundström B, Månson JC, Eklund G, Pettersson F, Day NE (1985a) Reduction in mortality from breast cancer after mass screening with mammography. Lancet I: 829–832

Tabár L, Gad A, Holmberg L, Ljungquist U (1985b) Significant reduction in advanced breast cancer. Results of the first seven years of mammography screening in Kopparberg, Sweden. Diagn Imag clin Med 54: 158–164

Tabár L, Gad A (1981) Screening for breast cancer: the Swedish trial. Radiology 138: 219–222

Verbeck ALM, Hendriks JHLC, Holland R, Mravunac M, Sturmans F, Day NE (1984) Reduction of breast cancer mortality through mass screening with modern mammography. Lancet I: 1222–1224

Screening for Breast Cancer in Malmö: A Randomized Trial

I. Andersson and B. F. Sigfússon

Department of Radiology, Malmö General Hospital, 21401 Malmö, Sweden

Study Design

The breast cancer screening program in Malmö was designed as a controlled study to investigate whether repeated invitation to screening with mammography might reduce the mortality from breast cancer. The program was started in January 1977 in the city of Malmö, which has about 235 000 residents. The invited cohort consisted of a 50% random sample of all women born between 1908 and 1932 (aged 45–69 years) living in the city at the time of the initiation of the screening. The randomization was done on an individual basis. Thus, the invited group and the control group were equally large, each consisting of approximately 21 000 women. The study is planned to go on for 10 years and will thus be finished in January 1987.

Technique

Film mammography is the single screening modality used. Thus, physical examination is not part of the screening procedure. In the first two screening rounds two views, the cranio-caudal and oblique views, were obtained. In the subsequent rounds either the oblique view only or both views were obtained depending on the parenchymal pattern as classified according to Wolfe; N1 and P1 breasts had the oblique view only, P2 and DY breasts both views. The mammographic technique has been described in more detail elsewhere (Andersson 1981).

The screening mammograms were classified as either suspicious for breast cancer or not. If considered suspicious, the patient was recalled for a complete mammogram. If the suspicion could be ruled out on the complete mammogram, the patient was informed immediately and sent home. If the suspicion persisted, the patient was referred to the team surgeon for further evaluation the same day.

Results and Comments

Almost five screening rounds have been completed as of June 1985. The interval between the rounds has been approximately 21 months on average. The data presented in the following are preliminary due to the fact that women who had a diagnosis of breast cancer after moving out of the city have not yet been traced.

The attendance rate was 74% in the first screening round and 70% in the subsequent rounds.

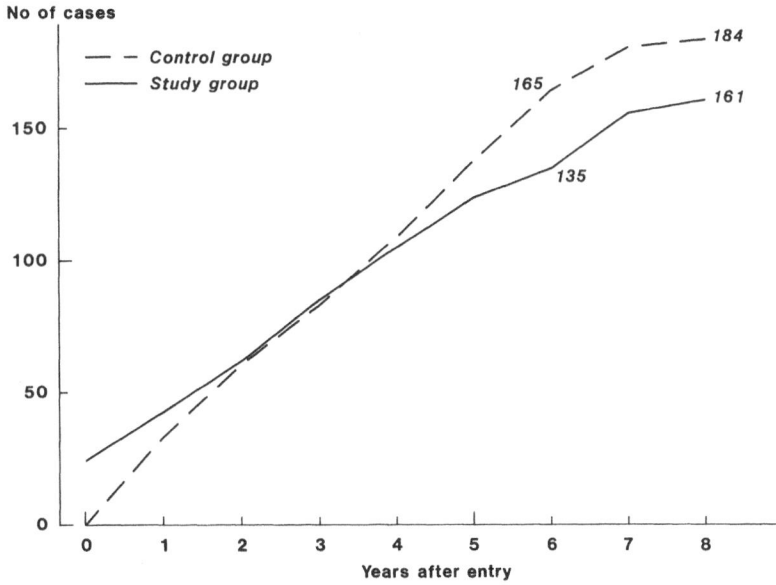

No of cases

— — Control group
——— Study group

184
165
161
135

Years after entry

Fig. 1. Cumulative number of patients with stage II–IV carcinoma

Through June 1985 breast cancer was found in 332 women at screening. Eighty-two women who were screened negative appeared with breast cancer in the intervals between screenings and 95 women who were invited but did not participate also appeared with cancer, which makes a total of 509 women with breast cancer in the invited group. This should be compared with 355 women with cancer in the control group during the same period. The excess number of women with cancer in the invited group originates mainly from the first screening round, in which 118 women with breast cancer were detected.

Figure 1 shows the cumulative number of stage II–IV cancers in the study and control groups. There was an excess of 24 stage II–IV cancers in the study group at the beginning of the program due to cases detected in the first screening round. Only after about 3 years did the number of stage II–IV cancers in the control group balance that in the study group. Then the trend has been an increasing difference in favor of the study group. At 6 years the difference was 30 cases, at 7 and 8 years about 24 cases, which means about 22% and 15% more stage II–IV cancers in the control group respectively. The reason why the curves level off at the end is that the entire population has not been followed for the whole period.

In Fig. 2 cases detected in the first screening round were excluded. The figure illustrates more clearly the impact of the screening program on the stage distribution after the prevalent screening.

In Fig. 3 the patients with stage II–IV cancer were stratified by age at entry into the study. It appears that the difference in favor of the invited group applies to the older women and there is no difference in the younger women.

In the period after the first screening the deficit of stage II carcinoma in the study group is more than balanced by an excess of stage I carcinoma (Fig. 4). The number of stage III and IV carcinomas is approximately the same in the study and control groups. Even excluding the first screening there is a slight excess in the total number of breast cancers in the study group. There are several possible explanations for this. On average the

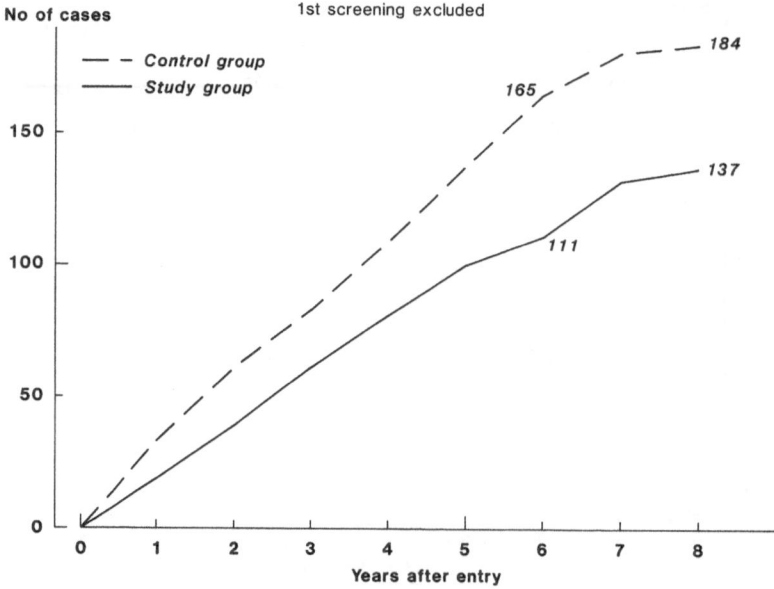

Fig. 2. Cumulative number of patients with stage II–IV carcinome, first screening excluded

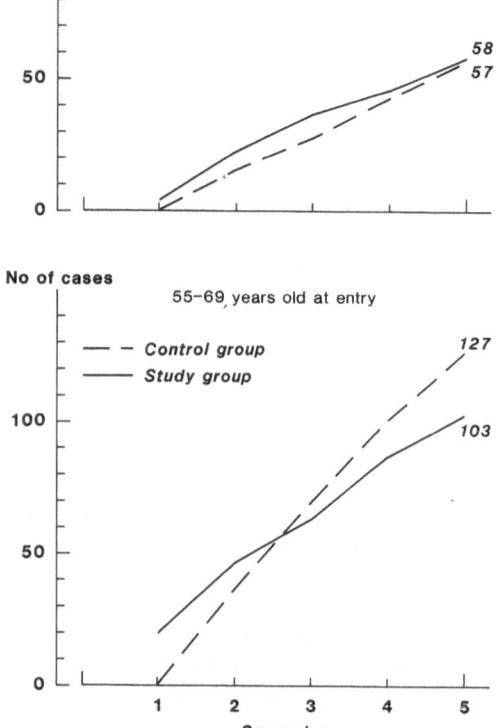

Fig. 3. Cumulative number of patients with stage II–IV carcinoma by age at entry

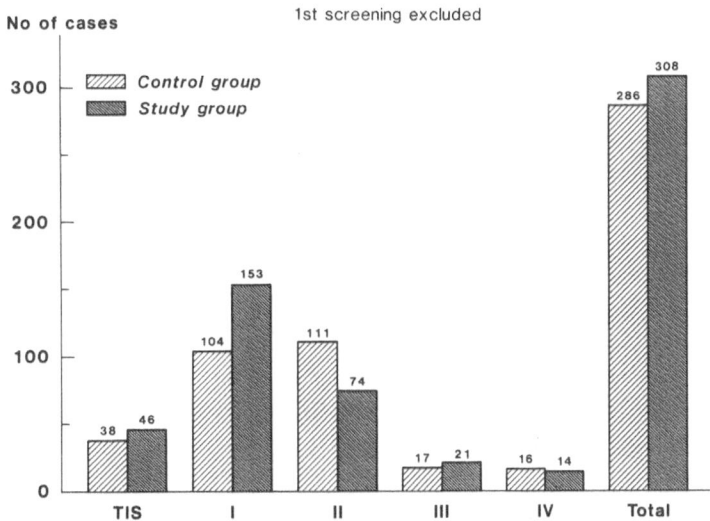

Fig. 4. Stage distribution by group through fourth screening, first screening excluded

breast cancer diagnosis is made later in the control group than in the study group, which might imply a reduced number of breast cancer cases in the control group due to death in intercurrent disease. Also, cancers that were detectable at the first screening but overlooked and detected later contribute to the excess.

The difference in the number of stage II–IV cancers between the invited group and control group is somewhat smaller than that reported from a similar study in Sweden in the counties of Kopparberg and Östergötland (Tabár et al. 1985). There are several possible explanations. One is the difference in participation rate which was higher in the Kopparberg-Östergötland study, 89% in the first and 83% in the second screening. This may reflect different attitudes to screening in the urban population in Malmö as compared with the mixed rural and urban population in the Kopparberg and Östergötland counties. From Fig. 5 it is clear that the group of nonparticipants contributed a substantial proportion of the stage II–IV cancers in Malmö. Many of these women had undoubtedly noted the mass in the breast already when they got the invitation to screening.

Another factor of importance is the availability of mammography in the community. If a large proportion of the control group women actually had mammography more or less as a screening procedure, it would also tend to reduce the difference between the invited group and control group.

To assess the importance of this factor a random sample of 250 control group women were checked for any mammographic examination during the period under investigation. It turned out that 14% had had one mammogram from the date of entry through June 1985, 4% had had two mammograms, and 6% had had three or more. Thus, although about 25% of the women had at least one mammogram relatively few women were examined on a regular basis.

The mammographic activities would also be reflected in the mechanism of case detection in the control group. Actually, 20% of the cancers in the control group were detected by mammography only and another 10% by routine physical examination. The latter group was not necessarily asymptomatic; however, many of these patients had symptoms primarily unrelated to the breasts.

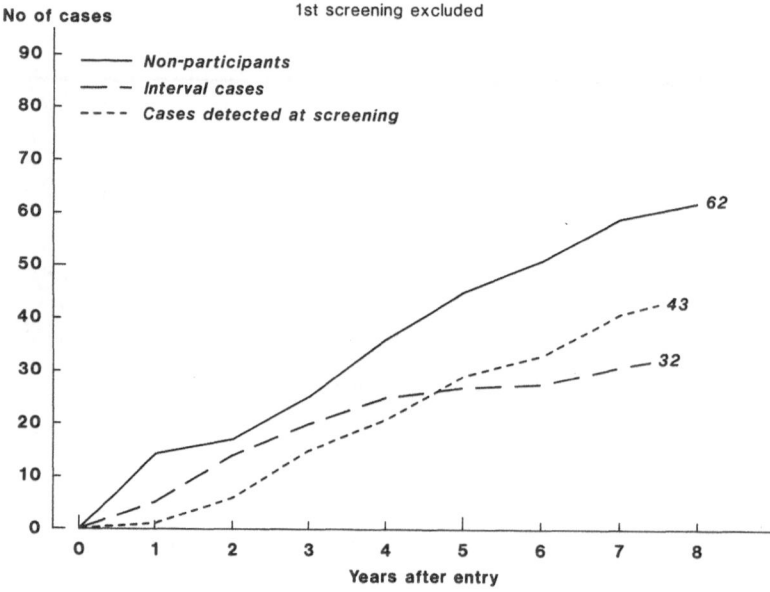

Fig. 5. Cumulative number of stage II–IV carcinomas in the study group, first screening excluded

A difference in the sensitivity of the screening procedure would be another possible explanation for our results as compared with the Kopparberg-Östergötland study. Factors influencing the sensitivity of mammography such as the parenchymal pattern of the breast may differ in different populations.

As mentioned above we have not yet traced those women who got a diagnosis of breast cancer after moving out of the city. There might well be more stage II–IV cancers belonging to the control group than to the invited group among these women. If so, that would increase the difference in favor of the study group.

It is important to underline that we do not exactly know how the difference in stage distribution reflects the future mortality. For example, we do not know if a stage II cancer detected at screening has the same prognosis as a stage II cancer in the control group.

In summary, we have documented a more favorable stage distribution in the study group than in the control group, indicating a future reduction of the breast cancer mortality as a result of screening. The magnitude of the effect on the mortality remains to be assessed. The effect of screening for breast cancer may vary with factors such as participation rate, number of the women in the control group undergoing mammography, and the sensitivity of the screening procedure.

References

Andersson I (1981) Radiographic screening for breast carcinoma. I. Program and primary findings in 45–69 year old women. Acta Radiol (Diagn) 22: 185–194

Tabár L, Fagerberg CJG, Gad A, Baldetorp L, Holmberg LH, Gröntoft O, Ljungquist U, Lundström B, Månsson JC, Eklund G, Day NE, Pettersson F (1985) Reduction in mortality from breast cancer after mass screening with mammography. Randomised trial from the Breast Cancer Screening Group of the Swedish National Board of Health and Welfare. Lancet 1: 829–832

The Guildford Breast Screening Project: 6-Year Assessment

B. A. Thomas and J. L. Price

Guildford Breast Screening Project, Jarvis Screening Centre, Stoughton Road, Guildford, Surrey, GU1 1LJ, United Kingdom

Introduction

The United Kingdom trial of methods for the early detection of breast cancer (TEDBC) was established in 1979 to study the impact of various early detection measures on the incidence, staging and mortality rate for breast cancer in eight trial populations; four populations act as controls, two have initiated breast self-examination programmes and two have screening programmes of annual clinical examination and biannual mammography. These populations consisted of some 23 000–25 000 women aged 45–64 years (at the start of the trial) registered with every primary care practitioner working in the Health Districts (UK Trial of Early Detection of Breast Cancer Group 1981) (Fig. 1).

There is no national age/sex register available for the United Kingdom and sampling suggests that these registers are at least 15% inaccurate, making acceptance rates for early detection measures appear low when compared with programmes with access to fully computerised updated registers.

This paper relates to the Guildford Project, which started screening in January 1979, the initial round being completed in March 1981. Women were entered into the trial when their screening invitation was sent. The projected seven screening rounds of the initial protocol should be completed in early 1987. Any one project study year therefore extends over 3 calendar years, when 1 year is allowed for follow-up, to include interval cancers and cancers in women who fail to attend for screening. In contrast the study years for the control populations consist of all cancer cases diagnosed in each calendar year, the women being registered in the project simultaneously on 1 January 1980 (Fig. 2). It should be noted that historic data for age-standardised mortality rates for the populations in the 10 years prior to the study showed a 10% lower average mortality rate in the control districts as compared with the two screening districts (UK Trial of Early Detection of Breast Cancer Group 1981).

The screening method consists of clinical examination by a specially trained doctor followed by single 45° oblique view mammography with the films being interpreted by the doctor who examined the woman, and a second opinion from the project radiologist, when appropriate.

One year later women who attend are recalled for clinical examination by a specially trained nurse. In the 3rd, 5th and 7th years, all women are reinvited to attend for full screening (clinical and mammogram), with a clinical examination alone repeated in years 4 and 6 for those who attended the previous screening round. The present progress of the screening rounds is indicated in Fig. 2 and full procedural details and preliminary results have been published previously (Thomas et al. 1983, 1984).

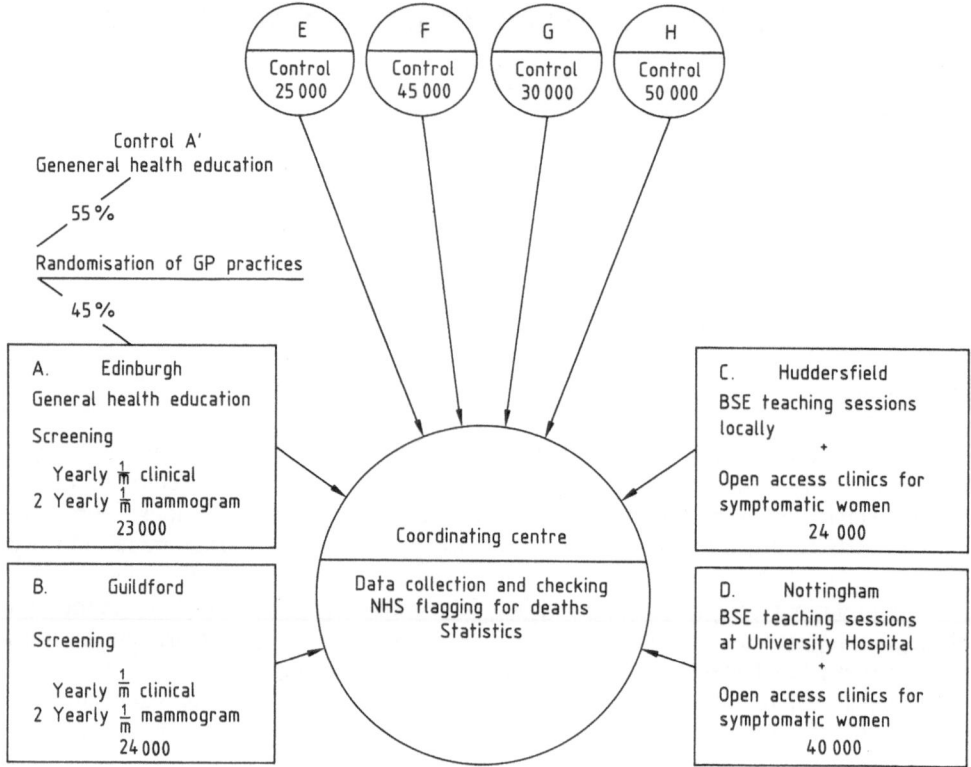

Fig. 1. United Kingdom trial of methods for the early detection of breast cancer

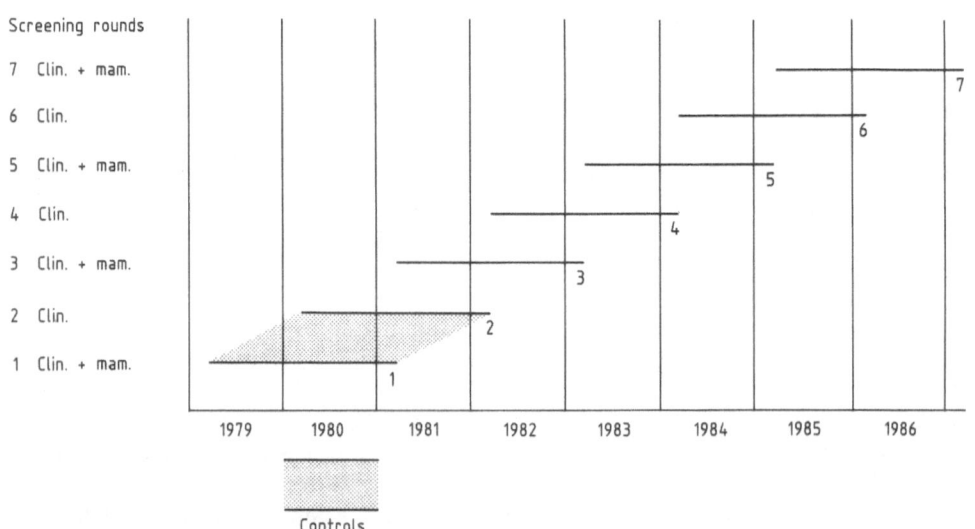

Fig. 2. Guildford Breast Screening Project: screening rounds and study years

Table 1. Guildford Breast Screening Project: original cohort

	1st Screen clin + mam	2nd Screen clin	3rd Screen clin + mam	4th Screen clin	5th Screen clin + mam	6th Screen (½) clin
Invited	24069	16356	21141	14206	19091	6645
Attended	16586	13940	14599	12572	13411	5820
%	69%	85%	69%	89%	70%	88%
Recall percentage of routine screened	8.8%	9.8%	5.3%	6.4%	4.9%	3.7%
Cancer/1000 attended	5.5	0.9	3.9	1.4	3.1	1.5
Benign biopsy/1000 attended	9.7	2.9	3.2	0.8	1.5	0.5

1985 – 3000 addresses unknown.
clin, clinical examination; *mam*, mammography.

Follow-up Report

The attendance rate (Table 1) has remained remarkably constant at around 70% (of the registered population not known to have left the district) for the major screening rounds when clinical examination and mammography is offered. The intervening screening rounds offer clinical examination alone to those women who attended the preceding round and some 85%–90% accept. By 1985 some 3000 women initially on the registers are known not to be at the registered address and work is progressing on tracing whether the women left the population before or during the trial, or remain at a different address. The inaccuracy of the registers is a major organisational problem.

In rescreening rounds the recall rate has remained around 5% of women screened. Women are recalled to special review clinics where specialist facilities are available for clinical assessment, mammography – including magnification mammography, ultrasound examination and fine needle aspiration cytology (Thomas et al. 1983). Referral for a surgical opinion is made when appropriate, and has resulted in a cancer to benign biopsy ratio of 1:2 in the initial screening round, falling to around 2:1 in the rescreening rounds.

Staging of Cancers in the Project Population

All cancers diagnosed during 1979–1984 in women of the initial cohort are indicated in Table 2. Bilateral or multiple primary cancers are categorised by the more advanced lesion. Less than one-third of all cancers are over 2 cm in size, as measured by the pathologist. Nodal status is indicated, though since axillary clearance and internal mammary node sampling is not carried out on all cases, full staging cannot be given.

The contribution of the different types of screening round, the interval cancers and cancers in women who fail to attend are illustrated in Fig. 3, with, for comparison, the size of those cancers diagnosed in project women between January 1979 and their date of entry into the trial.

It will be noted that interval cancers are relatively few in number compared with "mammogram only" screening programmes, but the cancers detected on the clinical ex-

Table 2. Guildford Breast Screening Project: initial cohort – total cancers diagnosed 1979–1984, incidence of nodal involvement relative to tumour size

	%	No.	Known nodes – ve	Known nodes + ve	Node + ve (% of total)	
33.8%	10.3	In situ	31	6	0	0
	6.0	1– 5 mm	18	6	0	0
	17.5	6–10 mm	53	17	3	5.7
34.4%	20.5	11–15 mm	62	23	11	17.7
	13.9	16–20 mm	42	20	10	23.8
31.8%	13.9	21–50 mm	42	13	16	38.1
	17.9	Advanced	54	0	39	72.2
		Total	302	85	79	26.2

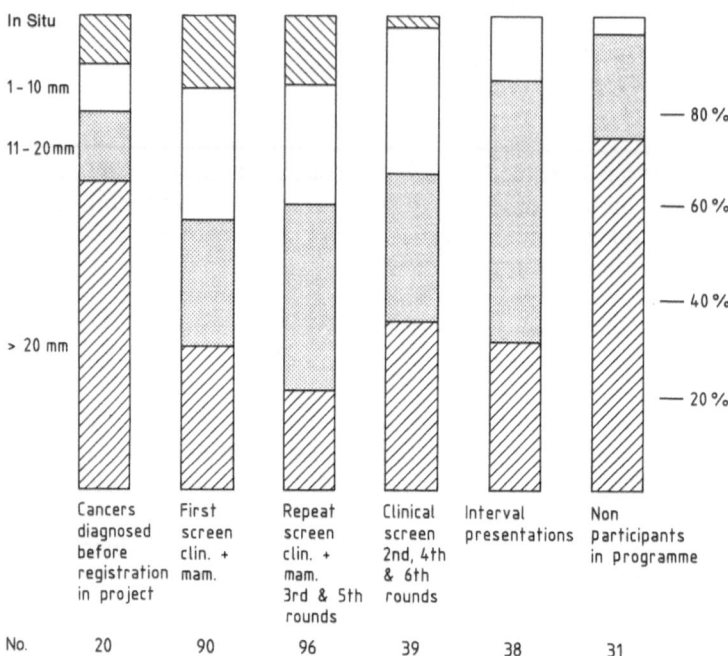

Fig. 3. Guildford Breast Screening Project: initial cohort January 1979–March 1985. Percentage distribution of cancers by presentation

amination 1 year after the full screening may be considered together with the interval cancers. The staging of these cancers diagnosed between mammographic screening rounds is encouraging with nearly two-thirds under 2 cm in diameter. Participation in a screening programme does seem to make women more "breast aware". Their willingness to report minor changes and the availability of facilities for their rapid investigation may well prove a major factor in determining the practical rescreening interval. Theoretical consideration of the apparent sensitivity of screening methods may well be altered significantly by the attitudes of the women concerned since any reluctance to take notice of or act upon minimal breast changes will result in a more advanced cancer being detected at the subsequent

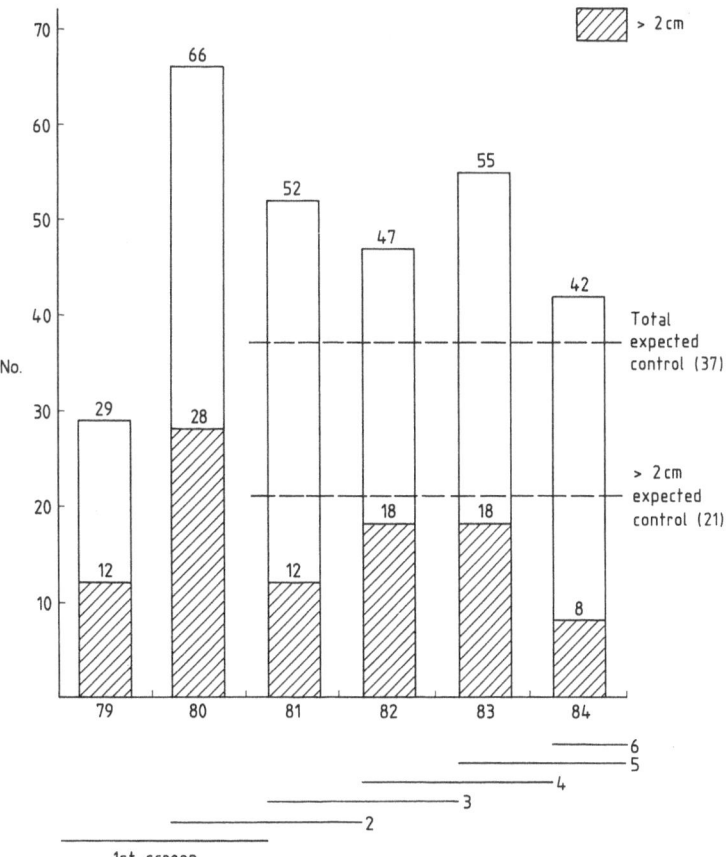

Fig. 4. Guildford Breast Screening Project: cancers diagnosed in the initial cohort 1979–1984. Numbers in the control groups are not yet available, but the expected figures are given based upon national figures

screening round. In these circumstances the screening method may appear to have a high sensitivity with few interval cancers but less favorable staging, while an encouragement of the minimally symptomatic appears to result in more interval cancers, a lower screening sensitivity but improved staging, and hopefully has a positive influence on mortality. Sensitivity of the screening method alone cannot therefore be necessarily used as an indicator to efficacy of a screening programme.

The distribution of the cancers detected in the programme in relation to calendar years is indicated in Fig. 4. While 1980 produced the highest workload for the hospital services, the implementation of the programme over a 2-year period otherwise has resulted in a relatively low workload, with total cancers having fallen now almost to the expected load in the control districts. There is a deficit of >2-cm cancers in the Guildford population subsequent to the initial screening round, which also has implications for treatment requirements.

No mortality data can be considered at this stage, but we are hopeful that the reduction in the rate of diagnosis of >2-cm cancers (Fig. 5) will precede a mortality reduction, as has been shown in the Swedish Trials (Tabar et al. 1985).

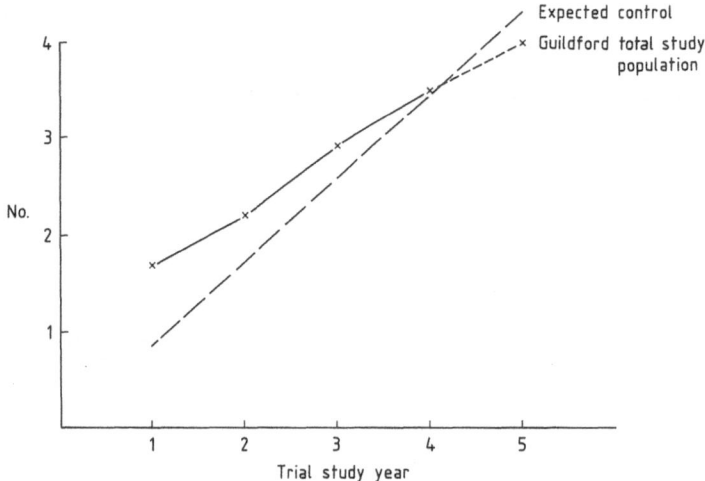

Fig. 5. Guildford Breast Screening Project: > 2-cm breast cancers/1000 woman years – initial cohort

References

Thomas BA et al. (1983) The guildford breast screening project. Clin Oncol 9: 121–129
Thomas BA et al. (1984) The first 3 years of the Guildford Breast Screening Project. In: Brünner S, Langfeldt B, Andersen PE (eds) Early detection of breast cancer. Springer, Berlin Heidelberg New York Tokyo, p 195 (Recent Results in Cancer Research, Vol 90)
UK Trial of Early Detection of Breast Cancer Group (1981) Description of Method

Mammography: Attitudes and Reactions*

S. Jakobsen, J. Beckmann, M. Beckmann, and S. Brünner

Department of Radiology, KAS Gentofte University Hospital, 2900 Hellerup,
Copenhagen, Denmark

Introduction

Since the Danish news media has demonstrated a long-term interest in breast cancer diagnosis and treatment, it can be assumed that the general public is well informed about both
the advantages and risk factors of mammography. Our study of women's current attitudes
toward mammography is an effort to predict the future acceptability of mammographic
screening.

In 1983 a consensus conference dealing with the subject of breast cancer diagnosis was
held in Copenhagen. The conclusion was that general screening of women for breast cancer should not be undertaken. This conference received considerable attention from the
news media.

A survey of women's attitudes toward mammography was carried out in Copenhagen
(Eliasen et al. 1981). It was of practical interest to us, therefore, to undertake a similar survey in 1984 to see if the news coverage of the 1983 conference had influenced women's attitudes toward mammography.

Material

Two groups of patients were studied. The first group consisted of 426 women who were referred to the Department of Diagnostic Radiology, Gentofte University Hospital, Copenhagen, for mammographic examination during the latter half of 1984. The average age of
this group was 43 years, ranging from 16 to 75 years. The second group consisted of
539 women, with an average age of 43 years, ranging from 16 to 82 years. Patients in this
group were referred to the X-Ray Department, Gentofte University Hospital, for examinations other than mammography, during the same period as the first group.

Information was gathered through patient completion of a questionnaire which was
distributed while the patients awaited examination.

Forty-six percent of the women referred to mammography, i.e., group I, performed
self-palpation at least once a month. In group II 30% of the women referred to other X-ray
examinations performed self-palpation at least once a month (Table 1). There is, therefore,
a connection between referral to mammography and regular examination of the breast.
Twenty-one percent of group I, as opposed to 33% of group II, seldom or never examined
their breasts. It is seen here that women who were not referred to mammography were less

---

* This study was carried out with the support of the Ib Henriksen Foundation.

Table 1. Self-examination

	Group I (mammography)		Group II (other examinations)	
Every week	5% (20) ⎫		3% (15) ⎫	
Several times a month	18% (75) ⎬ 46%		10% (54) ⎬ 30%	
Once a month	23% (96) ⎭		17% (90) ⎭	
Three to four times a year	31% (133)		33% (178)	
About once a year	14% (58) ⎫ 21%		21% (113) ⎫ 33%	
Never	7% (28) ⎭		12% (67) ⎭	

Table 2. How important?

	1984				1981
	Group I (mammography)		Group II (other examinations)		(mammography)
Very important	56% (240) ⎫ 90%		76% (412) ⎫ 87%		71% (212) ⎫ 97%
Important	34% (146) ⎭		11% (60) ⎭		26% (77) ⎭
Less important	2% (10)		2% (9)		1% (4)
Unnecessary	(1)		(2)		(0)
Don't know	4% (16)		4% (19)		2% (6)
Not answered	3% (13)		7% (37)		(1)

preoccupied with the risk of breast cancer, since they examined their breasts less frequently.

When asked if they attended regular control examinations by their physician, 45% of group I and 30% of group II answered "yes." As expected, regular control examinations of the breast occurred more frequently among women referred to mammography.

Both in 1981 and 1984, patients were asked about what importance they attached to mammography. How did they perceive its use regarding decisions on possible treatment or conjunction with symptoms such as palpable tumors, secretions, or breast pain. Table 2 shows that when the answer "important" and "very important" are compared, there seems to be no great difference between the two groups.

Asked in 1984 if they would consult another doctor, if their own physician refused to refer them to mammography, 66% of group I and 79% of group II answered affirmatively, as opposed to only 55% in 1981.

When asked if they were afraid of injury due to the radiation associated with mammography (Table 3), 72% of group I answered that they did not consider the examination to be dangerous, or only slightly so. Eight percent regarded mammography as a potentially dangerous examination. In group II, 64% felt that mammography was not dangerous, or only slightly so, while 12% considered it to be dangerous.

Patients have a high regard for the reliability of mammography (Table 4). When asked how reliable they felt mammography was in determining whether a lesion was malignant or benign, 54% of group I and 49% of group II answered "reliable" or "very reliable." The reliability question was not included in the 1981 study.

When asked if they would be afraid of the possible result of the mammography (Table 5), 67% of group I and 72% of group II answered that they would be only "slightly"

Table 3. Fear of radiation

	1984		1981
	Group I (mammography)	Group II (other examinations)	(mammography)
Very dangerous	(1)	2% (9)	2% (6)
Dangerous	8% (35)	10% (56)	13% (39)
Less dangerous	55% (233) ⎫ 72%	53% (283) ⎫ 64%	45% (135) ⎫ 58%
Not dangerous	17% (72) ⎭	11% (59) ⎭	13% (38) ⎭
Don't know	18% (77)	19% (102)	26% (78)
Not answered	2% (8)	6% (30)	1% (4)

Table 4. Reliability of mammography

	Group I (mammography)	Group II (other examinations)
Very reliable	13% (55)	10% (55)
Reliable	41% (173)	39% (211)
Less reliable	19% (80)	16% (86)
Unreliable	8% (34)	11% (60)
Don't know	17% (74)	20% (107)
Not answered	4% (20)	6% (30)

or "not at all" afraid of the result. In 1981, the figures were different. At that time, 36% of the women were "anxious" or "very anxious," only 28% were "not anxious," and 35% responded "don't know."

Discussion

Before discussing the data from our study, it is important to note some previously observed psychosocial characteristics of women in relation to their reactions to breast self-examination (Beckmann 1984; Greer et al. 1979). Women who demonstrate interest in breast self-examination tend to be:

1. Active participants in other disease prevention programs
2. Consult their physicians as soon as any breast cancer symptoms are suspected
3. Have a positive outlook regarding the diagnosis, treatment, and cure of breast cancer.

On the other hand, women who refuse to participate in breast self-examination tend to be:

1. Afraid that a cancer will actually be found
2. Fearful that such a finding will destroy their life
3. Feel that they should not go looking for more problems than they already have.

As background for our study, it should additionally be noted that the Danish Society for the Prevention of Cancer has maintained an intensive campaign to encourage women to examine their own breasts by self-palpation.

The psychological aspects of women who regularly carry out breast self-examination are similar to those seen in women who voluntarily participate in breast screening programs (Baines 1983; Gästrin 1981). We were, therefore, interested in knowing how many of these women performed self-examination regularly.

Our examination showed that less than half of the women in both groups, in spite of the extensive public information campaign in existence, made the recommended monthly self-palpation of the breast.

Twenty-one percent of the women in group II stated that they "seldom" or "never" examined their breasts for tumors. In light of this statistic, it is not surprising that many cases of breast cancer are discovered and treated too late.

As seen in Table 2, the two groups are almost the same regarding their views on mammographic examinations.

It seems interesting, however, that while 76% of group II found mammography "very important," only 56% of those who had actually been referred to mammography found it so. Perhaps the fact that the women had already been referred reduced the importance factor in their answer.

If a woman's own physician refuses to refer her to mammography, it seems that she is now more inclined to take the responsibility for the way in which her symptoms are investigated by finding another physician. Perhaps women have begun to lose faith in the authority of others to decide such things for them.

Comparison of group I's answers to the results of the 1981 survey demonstrates that the consensus conference, with all its media coverage, has not significantly influenced patients' attitudes regarding the risks associated with mammography (Table 3). Before the conference, 58% of the patients considered X-ray procedures "safe" or involving only "slight risk," as opposed to 72% in the present study. This implies that an increasing number of patients consider the radiation risks associated with mammography to be negligible.

Most women experience the suspected presence of breast cancer as a direct and real threat to their life, female identity, sexuality, and their domestic and marital relationships. It is natural, therefore, that a woman reacts with fear when there is a suspicion of breast cancer present. Fear of the result of the examination may prevent some women from undergoing mammography (Pitman 1974).

The increased amount of information that has been available to the public over the past 3 years has had a beneficial psychological effect (Table 5). There has been a decrease in fear of the result of the mammographic examination. Our survey results indicate that solid, trustworthy, and comprehensive information about a disease reduces the general level of apprehension associated with it.

Table 5. Fear of the result of the examination

| | 1984 | | 1981 |
	Group I (mammography)	Group II (other examinations)	(mammography)
Very anxious	6% (30) ⎫ 27%	11% (60) ⎫ 24%	7% (20) ⎫ 36%
Anxious	21% (89) ⎭	13% (69) ⎭	29% (86) ⎭
A little anxious	50% (213) ⎫ 67%	43% (233) ⎫ 72%	
Not anxious	17% (72) ⎭	29% (158) ⎭	28% (88)
Don't know	3% (12)	7% (39)	35% (104)
Not answered	2% (10)	2% (10)	2% (5)

Table 6. Would you participate in mammographic mass-screening?

	Yes	No	Don't know	Not answered
Group I (mammography)	84% (358)	4% (16)	7% (28)	6% (24)
Group II (other examinations)	83% (448)	4% (22)	9% (49)	4% (20)

The results from mammographic screening programs in Sweden (Andersson 1980; Tabár et al. 1985) and the Netherlands (Hendriks 1982) are useful. It will be interesting to create a similar mammographic screening program in Denmark, where it seems that the female population is interested in such a project (Table 6), with 84% of group I and 83% in group II indicating that they would participate in a mammographic mass screening. These numbers compare positively with actual Swedish mammographic screening in cities such as Malmö (Andersson 1980) and in county districts such as Kopparberg (Tabár et al. 1985), where participation levels of 75% and 85% were recorded.

Conclusion

Despite the general debate in the news media after a consensus conference in Denmark on radiation risks and the known disadvantages of mammography as an examination, most women today are well disposed toward mammographic screening. They consider mammography to be safe, or to involve only a slight risk. Most women would, therefore, probably participate in a countrywide mammographic screening program.

References

Andersson I (1981) Mammographic screening for breast carcinoma. Appearance of carcinoma and number of projections to be used at screening. Acta Radiol Diagn 2: 407-420

Baines CJ (1983) Some thoughts on why women do not do breast self-examination. Can Med Assoc J 128: 255-256

Beckmann J (1984) Aspects psychologiques des investigations de masse pour dépistage du cancer du sein. Int J Breast Mammary Pathol – Senologia 1983-1984, 2, 4: 219-221

Consensus-report (1983) Early detection of breast cancer. Danish Medical Research Council and Danish Hospital Institute. Tekst og Tryk A/S Vedbæk (in Danish)

Eliasen B, Dissing I, Brünner S (1981) Attitudes to and expectations of mammography among 300 women submitted to this investigation. Ugeskr Læger 143: 2306-2308

Gästrin G (1981) Breast cáncer control. Almquist and Wiksell International, Stockholm

Greer S, Morris T, Pettinggale KW (1979) Psychological responses to breast cancer. Lancet 2: 785-787

Hendriks JHCL Population screening for breast cancer by means of mammography in Nijmegen 1975-1980. Thesis 1982, Nijmegen

Pitman NJ (1974) Women's attitudes regarding breast cancer. Occupational Health Nursing 22: 20-23

Tabár L, Gad A, Holmberg LH et al. (1985) Reduction in mortality from breast cancer after mass screening with mammography. Lancet 1: 829-832

Mammography Screening:
Published Guidelines and Actual Practice

S. A. Feig

Department of Radiology, Thomas Jefferson University Hospital, Philadelphia, PA 19107, USA

By midsummer 1975, the future of mammography screening in the United States seemed assuredly successful. The 29 nationwide centers of the American Cancer Society-National Cancer Institute (ACS-NCI)-sponsored Breast Cancer Detection Demonstration Project (BCDDP) had been in operation since 1973. They had enrolled 280000 asymptomatic women aged 35–74 years for annual screening by mammography and physical examination for four successive years (Baker 1982). Recruitment of women into the project was excellent due in part to media attention given to the wife of the President of the United States, Mrs. Gerald Ford, and the wife of the Vice President, Mrs. Nelson Rockefeller, both of whom were successfully treated for breast cancer.

In September 1975, mammography screening suddenly became a national controversy when Dr. John Bailar, editor of the Journal of the National Cancer Institute, called public attention to the potential radiation risks. He subsequently expressed these concerns in medical journals (Bailar 1976, 1977, 1978). While conceding that for women above age 50 or 60, "the radiation risk may be small in relation to the expected benefit," he concluded that "the routine use of mammography in screening asymptomatic women may eventually take almost as many lives as it saves." His conclusions were not based on BCDDP data but rather on the higher radiation doses and lower mammographic detection rates for women enrolled in screening at the Health Insurance Plan of New York (HIP) during the 1960s (Feig 1979). These statements and their repercussions created a national hysteria. As a result, the BCDDP discontinued routine mammography screening of women under 50 years of age in 1977 (Culliton 1977 a, b; National Institutes of Health/National Cancer Institute 1978).

Screening Guidelines

In response to these concerns, the American College of Radiology (ACR) issued its first mammography screening guidelines (American College of Radiology 1976). These recommended "a baseline study between age 35 and 40, subsequent examinations at 1–3 year intervals between age 40 and 50, and annual or other regular interval examination after age 50". A chronological list of these and other guidelines issued from 1976 to 1986 may be found in Table 1.

In 1977, the NCI formally issued restrictions for the use of mammography at the BCDDP (Statement on Recommendations of the Consensus Development Panel on Breast Cancer Screening 1978). Between age 35–39, mammography could be performed only if there was a personal history of breast cancer or an abnormal physical examination. For women age 40–49, the history of breast cancer in a mother or sister was added to these

Table 1. A chronological list of guidelines for screening mammography

Year issued	Organization
1976	American College of Radiology
1977	National Cancer Institute
1977	American Cancer Society
1979	American College of Obstetricians and Gynecologists
1980	American Cancer Society
1981	American Academy of Family Physicians
1982	American Cancer Society
1982	American College of Radiology
1983	American Cancer Society
1984	American Medical Association
1985	American College of Physicians
1986	National Council on Radiation Protection and Measurements

indications. All women above age 50 were allowed to have annual mammograms. Although screening at the BCDDP was completed in 1981 (Baker 1982), these restrictions represent NCI's current recommendations to physicians and patients and are available in public information pamphlets (National Cancer Institute 1983, 1985).

Because the BCDDP was jointly supported by the ACS and NCI, the American Cancer Society in 1977 had to endorse the NCI recommendations (American Cancer Society 1980). In 1980 when the BCDDP was nearing completion, the ACS issued new recommendations based on the lower radiation dose and improved detection sensitivity, particularly among women below age 50, of the BCDDP compared with the HIP project (Feig 1979). The ACS advised a baseline mammogram for all women between age 35–40 and annual screening after age 50. Women between age 40 and 50 were not offered specific recommendations but rather advised to "consult their personal physician about the need for mammography in their individual cases" (American Cancer Society 1980).

The American College of Obstetricians and Gynecologists (ACOG) issued a mammography policy statement in 1979 which was amended in 1980. Even more than the ACS's statement, the ACOG policy left the frequency of examination up to the discretion of the individual physician. Clinical signs and symptoms of breast disease such as "masses or nipple discharge, lumps felt by the patient but not confirmed by physician palpation" and risk factors such as "previous diagnosis of breast cancer, family history of breast cancer in mother or sister, first pregnancy after age 30 and abnormal patterns in baseline mammogram suggestive of increased risk" were considered "indicators for mammograms in women of any age." A baseline study was advised between age 35 and 50. It was suggested that the "physician should determine the frequency of subsequent mammography from results of the baseline and other breast examinations. "Women over 50 were advised to receive regular breast examinations including mammography at intervals to be determined by the physician" (American College of Obstetricians and Gynecologists 1980). These guidelines are presently under review by an ACOG task force established in 1985.

The mammography guidelines from the American Academy of Family Physicians, issued in 1981, were also indefinite in suggesting screening intervals for women below age 50. A baseline study was urged for all women over 35. Examination of asymptomatic high-risk women under 50 years of age "at appropriate intervals" based on risk factors was urged. Annual examination of women over 50 years of age was advocated (American Academy of Family Physicians 1981).

Because of accumulating data on benefits gained by earlier detection, the American College of Radiology (ACR) prepared a more current version of its guidelines in 1982. These contained several changes from the previous 1976 ACR statement. The new guidelines advised "a first or baseline mammogram by age 40 with an earlier age preferable when there is a personal history of breast cancer or a history of pre-menopausal breast cancer in the patient's mother and/or sisters." The earlier statement had recommended "a baseline between age 35-40." The most important innovation was the recommendation "subsequent mammographic examination ... at 1-2 year intervals determined by the combined analysis of physical and mammographic findings and other risk factors, unless medically indicated sooner" for women age 40-50. Thus, the screening interval for these younger women had been shortened from the 1-3 year period listed in the earlier statement. In addition, the recommendation for women over age 50 was now for "annual mammography" in contrast to the less specific 1976 recommendation for "annual or other regular interval mammography" (American College of Radiology 1982).

Impelled by the 1982 ACR guidelines as well as reported results from the BCDDP which suggested that favorable benefit/risk ratios could be expected from screening women beginning at age 40 (Seidman 1977), the American Cancer Society in 1983 modified its guidelines to recommend that mammography be performed at intervals of 1-2 years in asymptomatic women age 40-49 years (American Cancer Society 1983).

It should be emphasized that both the ACR and ACS guidelines stress the need for periodic breast self-examination and physical examination as well as mammography. The ACR states that "all women should be taught proper breast self-examination by age 20 and should have an annual physical examination of the breasts after age 35" (American College of Radiology 1982). The ACS advises monthly breast self-examination after age 20 and physical examination every 3 years from age 20 to 40 and annually after age 40 (American Cancer Society 1980).

The 1983 ACS guidelines seemed to herald a growing consensus in the medical community regarding the efficacy of screening mammography of asymptomatic women beginning before age 40. In 1984, the American Medical Association Council on Scientific Affairs issued a report entitled "Early Detection of Breast Cancer," which stated that "physicians should recognize the importance of mammography as an effective screening device to detect early breast cancer." The report contained the following recommendations based on the ACR and ACS guidelines: "Ideally, the first or baseline mammogram should be obtained by age 35 to 40 years. An earlier age is recommended when there is a personal history of breast cancer or a history of pre-menopausal breast cancer in a patient's mother or sister. Subsequently, screening mammograms from age 40 through 49 years should be performed at one- to two-year intervals at the discretion of the patient's physician, depending on the combined analysis of physical and mammographic findings and other risk factors. Annual mammography is now recommended for all women aged 50 and older" (American Medical Association 1984).

One significant exception to the favorable trend toward mammography screening was the breast cancer screening position paper issued in 1985 by the American College of Physicians, the organization of physicians engaged in the practice of internal medicine (American College of Physicians 1985). The report stated that it "cannot conclude that adequate data are available to decide that asymptomatic women between the ages of 40 and 49 should receive annual screening mammograms." The committee felt that more direct indication of the effect of screening on mortality reduction among these younger women was necessary. The paper also expressed concern regarding potential radiation risks, unnecessary surgery from false-positive results, and the costs and feasibility of widespread implementation.

Accordingly, the American College of Physicians advised mammography screening among women age 40–49 only if there was a personal or close family history of breast cancer or if breast self-examination or physician examination were technically difficult. The position paper supported screening women age 50–59 but did not suggest the frequency of examination. They also questioned the advisability of screening women between age 60 and 69 and deferred such a decision to the clinical judgment of the individual physician until more data are available.

The most recent pronouncement on mammography screening is that of the NCRP (National Council on Radiation Protection and Measurements 1986). Based on a quantitative comparison of projected benefits and risks, the Council concluded that "annual mammographic examinations appear to provide favorable benefit-risk ratios in women age 40 or above if acceptable image quality is maintained with an average glandular dose for the two-view examination of each breast of 0.8 rad or less. Two-view doses of up to 0.2 rad ... result in a favorable benefit-risk ratio for women, even below age 40."

Rates of Compliance

Despite a substantial increase in the number of mammographic studies performed in the United States over the past 5–10 years, only a small proportion of women in the breast cancer age group receive screening. Among physicians responding to recent polls, only 4%–17% refer women over age 50 for annual screening (Bassett et al. 1985; Battista 1983; Cohen et al. 1982; Cummings et al. 1983; Dietrich and Goldberg 1984). However, since many women do not see a physician at least once a year, the actual percentage of women above age 50 being screened may be lower than indicated by these studies.

A recent national survey indicated that 11% of all physicians, 9% of general practitioners and internists, and 17% of gynecologists follow or exceed the ACS guidelines for screening all women above age 35 (American Cancer Society 1985).

A poll of Los Angeles physicians found that gynecologists and surgeons are more likely to refer patients for screening than general practitioners and internists. Younger physicians are more likely to advise screening than older ones. Among the Los Angeles physicians, 19% of those under age 40 but only 9.5% of those over age 40 refer women age 50 and above for annual mammography (Bassett et al. 1985).

One study of family physicians in New York State investigated screening referrals for women above versus below age 50. For women 41–50 years, screening was recommended every year by 3% and once every 2 years by 10%. For women over 50 years, screening was recommended every year by 8% and once every 2 years by 14% (Cummings et al. 1983). Although more women above age 50 were being screened than those age 40–50, ACS screening guidelines were followed more often in the 40–50 year age group.

Physicians are much less likely to advise mammography than other screening procedures. Physician compliance with ACS screening guidelines was reported as 11% for mammography, 80% for breast physical examination, and 70% for the Pap test (American Cancer Society 1985).

Thus, patients are less likely to receive mammography than other screening studies. Among Michigan women, 69% of those age 35–49 and 57% of those age 50–64 practice monthly breast self-examination. For those age 40 and older, 70% receive annual physical examination of the breasts. However, only 22% of the 40- to 49-year-olds and 25% of women older than 50 underwent at least a baseline and one follow-up mammogram (Fox et al. 1985).

Reasons for Noncompliance

The major reasons for physician noncompliance seem to be the high cost of the mammographic procedure, the relatively low yield of cancers detected, the perceived ineffectiveness of early detection, and concern about possible radiation risk. Among physicians surveyed who did not completely agree with the ACS guidelines, 39% felt mammography was too expensive, 33% were concerned that it exposed the patient to too much radiation, 28% thought that it was unnecessary to perform annually, 14% said there was no need to screen patients in the absence of a family history of breast cancer, and 16% believed the yield was too low (American Cancer Society 1985).

Of the Los Angeles physicians who did not refer asymptomatic patients for mammography, 55% cited the high cost and low yield and only 7.3% were primarily concerned about the radiation hazard (Bassett et al. 1985).

Family physicians from New York State, when asked about the major deterrent for not recommending screening mammography, mentioned concern about radiation risk (43%), low probability of detecting cancer through screening (33%), unacceptably high cost (23%), and unreliable results (21%) (Cummings et al. 1983).

Physicians in Ottawa mentioned the perceived ineffectiveness of the procedure (51%), concern about radiation risk (28%), and nonaccessibility to service (10%) (Battista 1983).

Among New York women enrolled in a breast and uterine screening program who did not comply with a referral for screening mammography, almost two-thirds cited concern about radiation as a principal reason for noncompliance (Lane and Fine 1983).

Methods for Increasing Compliance

It would seem that better education of patients and physicians is needed to increase the level of screening. In one study, 80% of Los Angeles physicians said that they would recommend annual screening upon a patient's request (Bassett et al. 1985). In another Los Angeles study, 93% of women said they would probably agree to screening mammography if advised by their physician (Reeder et al. 1980). Thus, the prevailing attitude toward screening seems to be one of inertia or mild reluctance rather than opposition.

Several attempts to increase screening referrals have been reported in the literature and have met with varying degrees of success. All were conducted within residency programs and included control group comparisons. The strategies utilized were computer reminders (8% for the intervention group vs. 2% for the controls) (McDonald et al. 1984), an educational seminar (9% vs. 3.5%) (Fox 1985 a, b), and face-sheet guidelines attached to the patient's chart (32% vs. 4%) (Cohen et al. 1982).

These studies suggest that substantial increases in the use of mammography may not come from limited interventional measures alone but also require a general medical consensus regarding the efficacy of screening and the presence of a strong mammography section in the individual hospital. There are many reasons to believe that the underuse of mammography results more from lack of acceptance by physicians than resistance from patients. If mammography screening is to be fully implemented, radiologists must not only educate clinicians but also maintain high technical and interpretive standards for the examination.

Examination cost may be another significant factor. In one study when a change in funding policy discontinued mammography payments for one-half of referrals, women whose mammography was paid for by the project had a higher rate of compliance (54%) than those who paid for the examination themselves (33%). The effect on compliance was greater among asymptomatic women and those with normal findings on physical examination (Lane and Fine 1983).

At present, the nation's largest health insurers such as Aetna Life and Casualty Insurance Company, Prudential Insurance Company, and the Blue Cross and Blue Shield Association do not cover routine preventive care examinations such as screening mammography. Most health care policy changes come about at the request of policy holders so that increased public awareness of the value of screening could effect such a change. On the other hand, policy holders could apply pressure on insurers to restrain premium cost increases rather than expand coverage. Employers, in the interest of controlling health care costs, often prefer to provide only basic insurance protection. Nevertheless, many observers predict that insurers will cover routine mammography screening soon. Blue Cross/ Blue Shield and ACS officials have been talking about developing such coverage (American Medical News 1986).

The Health Insurance Plan of Greater New York (HIP), a health maintenance organization, which provides total health care coverage using its own physicians, has included screening mammography coverage for many years. Recently, the Health Maintenance Organization of New Jersey/Pennsylvania (HMO-PA/NJ) decided to provide screening mammography coverage for all women policy holders (FitzGerald 1986).

It is also possible that an increase in screening mammography could result from the malpractice crisis in the United States. Failure to diagnose breast cancer is generating a growing number of professional liability actions against physicians. The increasing likelihood of a lawsuit from failure to diagnose breast cancer, along with steadily rising costs of professional liability insurance, may pressure physicians to comply with screening guidelines. A physician may be liable if he does not follow the ACS screening guidelines. As of 1 January 1986, Colorado physicians covered by the Colorado Physicians Insurance Company (COPIC) who are involved in breast cancer malpractice claims will face a surcharge of up to $ 25 000 and possible cancellation of their insurance if they fail to observe the American Cancer Society guidelines in treating suing patients. Professional liability companies in other states will be watching the Colorado experiment closely (American Medical News 1986).

References

American Academy of Family Physicians (1981) Mammography guidelines developed by the AAFP Committee on Cancer. AAFP Reporter 8, 1: 15
American Cancer Society (1980) Cancer of the breast (In) guidelines for the cancer-related checkup, recommendations and rationale. CA 30: 224–232
American Cancer Society (1982) Mammography 1982: a statement of the American Cancer Society. CA 32: 226–230
American Cancer Society (1983) Mammography guidelines 1983: Background statement and update of cancer-related checkup guidelines for breast cancer detection in asymptomatic women age 40–49. CA 33: 255
American Cancer Society (1985) Survey of physicians' attitudes and practices in early cancer detection. CA 35: 197–213
American College of Obstetrics and Gynecology (1980) Mammography statement. Washington DC
American College of Physicians, Health and Public Policy Committee (1985) The use of diagnostic tests for screening and evaluating breast lesions. Ann Intern Med 103: 143–146

American College of Radiology (1976) Policy statement on mammography. ACR Bulletin 32: 1-2

American College of Radiology (1982) Guidelines for mammography. ACR Bulletin 38: 6-7

American Medical Association, Council on Scientific Affairs (1984) Early detection of breast cancer. JAMA 252: 3008-3011

American Medical Association (1986) Failure to diagnose breast cancer, hot topic. American Medical News, Feb 28, 1986, pp 3, 19-20, 22

Baker LH (1982) Breast cancer detection demonstration project: five-year summary report. CA 32: 194-225

Bailar JC (1976) Mammography: a contrary view. Ann Intern Med 84: 77-84

Bailar JC (1977) Screening for early breast cancer: pros and cons. Cancer 39: 2783-2795

Bailar JC (1978) Mammography screening: a reappraisal of benefits and risks. Clin Obstet Gynecol 21: 1-14

Bassett LW, Bunnell DH, Cerny JA, et al. (1985) Screening mammography: a survey of 4,200 referring physicians. Radiology 157 (P): 53

Battista RN (1983) Adult cancer prevention in primary care: patterns of practice in Quebec. Am J Public Health 73: 1036-1039

Cohen DI, Littenberg B, Wetzel C, et al. (1982) Improving physician compliance with preventive medicine guidelines. Medical Care 20: 1040-1045

Culliton BJ (1977a) Cancer Institute unilaterally issues new restrictions on mammography. Science 196: 853-857

Culliton BJ (1977b) Mammography controversy: NIH's entree into evaluating technology. Science 198: 171-173

Cummings KM, Funch DP, Mettlin C, et al. (1983) Family physicians' beliefs about breast cancer screening by mammography. J Fam Pract 17: 1029-1034

Dietrich AJ, Goldberg H (1984) Preventive content of adult primary care: do generalists and subspecialists differ? Am J Public Health 74: 223-227

Feig SA (1979) Low-dose mammography: application to medical practice. JAMA 242: 2107-2109

FitzGerald S (1986) HMO will begin offering free screening for cancer. The Philadelphia Inquirer April 24, pp 1A, 13A

Fox S, Tsou CV, Klos DS (1985a) Increasing mammography screening: an application of general principles of CME methodology. J Psychosomatic Obstet Gynecol 4: 95-104

Fox S, Tsou CV, Klos DS (1985b) An intervention to increase mammography screening by residents in family practice. J Fam Pract 20: 467-471

Fox S, Baum JK, Klos DS, et al. (1985) Breast cancer screening: the underuse of mammography. Radiology 156: 607-611

Lane DS, Fine HL (1983) Compliance with mammography referrals. Implications for breast cancer screening. New York State J Med 83: 173-176

McDonald CJ, Hui SL, Smith DM, et al. (1984) Reminders to physicians from an introspective computer medical record. Ann Intern Med 100: 130-138

National Cancer Institute (1983) Breast cancer: we're making progress every day. NIH Publication No 83-2409. US Department of Health and Human Services, Public Health Service, National Institutes of Health, National Cancer Institute, Bethesda, MD

National Cancer Institute (1985) Breast Exams. What you should know. NIH Publication No 85-2000, US Department of Health and Human Services, Public Health Service, National Institutes of Health, National Cancer Institute, Bethesda, MD

National Council on Radiation Protection and Measurements (1986) NCRP Report No 85: mammography - a user's guide. NCRP, Bethesda, MD, pp 114-127

National Institutes of Health/National Cancer Institute (1978) National Cancer Institute Consensus Development Meeting on Breast Cancer Screening. Issues and recommendations. JNCI 60: 1519-1521

Reeder S, Berkanovic E, Marcus AC (1980) Breast cancer detection behavior among urban women. Public Health Reports 95: 276-281

Seidman H (1977) Screening for breast cancer in younger women, life expectancy gains and losses: an analysis according to risk indicator groups. CA 27: 66-87

Statement on recommendations of the Consensus Development Panel on Breast Cancer Screening (1978) JNCI 1523-1524

Projected Benefits and Risks from Mammographic Screening

S. A. Feig

Department of Radiology, Thomas Jefferson University Hospital, Philadelphia, PA 19107, USA

Results from recent studies can be used to compare the benefits and risks of mammographic screening with more accuracy than previously possible. Estimates for the theoretical risk from current low-dose mammography can be derived from populations exposed to high doses of radiation. A reasonable range of values for the benefit from mammographic screening can be obtained from combined analysis of recent screening projects.

Estimation of Risk

It is not known if a mean breast dose of 0.1 rad for screen-film mammography or 0.5 rad for xeromammography (Stanton et al. 1984) increases breast cancer risk. However, excess breast cancers have been found in populations exposed to considerably higher doses of 100–2000 rad. These include Japanese A-bomb survivors (Tokunaga et al. 1979), North American women receiving multiple chest fluoroscopies for tuberculosis (Boice and Monson 1977; Howe 1984), and American and Swedish women treated with radiotherapy for benign breast disease (Shore et al. 1977; Baral et al. 1977).

If there is a risk from low doses, these studies indicate that it does not occur until at least 10 years postexposure, but may last for the patient's remaining lifetime. The high-dose studies can also provide an indirect estimate for low-dose risk.

The magnitude of low-dose risk will depend on the dose-response model chosen to make this estimation (Fig. 1). If risk per rad remains constant regardless of dose, then 1 rad

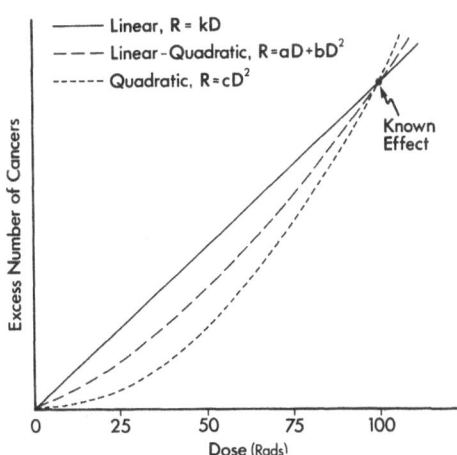

Fig. 1. Models for possible dose-response relation at low doses

would convey 1/100th the risk of 100 rad. This linear relationship between high- and low-dose risk occurs in a minority of radiation-induced animal tumors. Although it may not hold for breast cancer in humans, it can define the upper limits of low-dose risk. Using this method, the National Cancer Institute, in 1977, estimated that such risk might be 3.5 excess breast cancers/10^6 women/year per rad for women exposed at age 35 years or older (Upton et al. 1977).

It is also possible that risk per rad is less at low doses where most radiation-induced animal tumors demonstrate a curvilinear (quadratic) dose response relationship (United Nations Scientific Committee on the Effects of Atomic Radiation 1972; Webster 1981). When this model is applied to humans, the risk per rad at low doses would be 1/100th that of a linear extrapolation, i. e., 0.035 excess breast cancers/10^6 women per year per rad. Another model for low-dose risk is the linear-quadratic (Committee on the Biological Effects of Ionizing Radiation 1980). Here, risk is half that of the linear model, i. e., 1.8 excess breast cancers/10^6 women per year per rad.

Until lately, no human study contained enough patients exposed at low doses to allow a clear choice among the three dose response models (Land et al. 1980). However, a recent study of Canadian sanatoria patients supports a quadratic rather than a linear, but cannot exclude a linear-quadratic relation (Howe 1984). Also, this study found no evidence of risk for women exposed above age 40. A similar observation has been made in a recent study of A-bomb survivors which found no excess risk among those above age 30 at time of exposure to 99 rad or less (Tokunaga et al. 1984). Thus, the risk from screening women above age 35 may be so negligible as to be almost nonexistent (Feig 1984).

Comparison of Benefit and Risk

Benefits and risks can be compared when expressed in similar terms such as years of life expectancy gained from screening versus years of life expectancy lost from radiation. A range of reasonable estimates for such values can be based on results of recent screening projects (Shapiro 1982; Feig 1979, 1984; Milbrath 1981; Tabár, this volume; Hendrix, this volume). In the absence of screening, the average breast cancer patient will lose years of life expectancy. The benefit from a single mammographic screening can be equated with a percentage reduction in the years of life expectancy lost from cancers that in the absence of screening would surface clinically during 1 year. Benefits from a 20%, 40%, or 60% reduction of such loss among 20000 women aged 40–49 and 50–59 are given in Tables 1 and 2.

These benefits can be compared with the years of life expectancy possibly lost from radiation (Tables 1, 2). A mean glandular dose of 0.1 rad from a two-view screen-film mammographic examination has been used (Stanton et al. 1984). Higher-dose methods might result in proportionately greater risks. Four methods of low-dose risk projection have been applied: no risk, quadratic, linear-quadratic, and linear.

Several conclusions can be drawn. First, benefits from screening women age 50–59 are 25% greater than those from screening women age 40–49. This is due to the higher breast cancer incidence in older women: 42/20000 vs. 26/20000, an effect which is partially offset by their shorter natural life expectancy: 27.2 years vs. 36.3 years.

Secondly, benefits considerably exceed risks for any combination considered. Even with a 20% reduction of life expectancy lost and linear risk projection at age 40–49, benefits exceed risk by 100/1. However, as previously indicated, a 40%–60% mortality reduction can be expected from screening women over age 50. Although the percentage mortal-

Table 1. Estimation of years of life expectancy gained/lost from single screening of 20000 women, age 40–49

Risk model	Reduction of years of life expectancy lost		
	20%	40%	60%
No risk	100/0	200/0	300/0
Quadratic	100/0.01	200/0.01	300/0.01
Linear-quadratic	100/0.5	200/0.5	300/0.5
Linear	100/1.0	200/1.0	300/1.0

1. Years of life expectancy lost for the average breast cancer patient age 40–49 in absence of screening = average life expectancy - average life expectancy for all invasive breast cancers (nonscreening) = 36.3 – 17.1 = 19.2. [Based on data from Life Tables of the United States 1900–2050 (1983) and Seidman (1977)]
2. Years of life expectancy gained = years of life expectancy lost in absence of screening × annual incidence × % reduction in loss = 19.2 × 26 × 20% or 40% or 60%. [Based on data from Seidman and Mushinski (1983)]
3. Risk based on a mean glandular dose of 0.1 rad and a linear risk of 3.5 cancers/10^6 women per year per rad. Life Expectancy Tables of the United States 1900–2050 (1983) were used to calculate the remaining population at risk.

Table 2. Estimation of years of life expectancy gained/lost from single screening of 20000 women, age 50–59

Risk model	Reduction of years of life expectancy lost		
	20%	40%	60%
No risk	125/0	250/0	375/0
Quadratic	125/0.004	250/0.004	375/0.004
Linear-quadratic	125/0.2	250/0.2	375/0.2
Linear	125/0.4	250/0.4	375/0.4

1. Years of life expectancy lost for the average breast cancer patient, age 50–59, in absence of screening = 27.2 – 12.3 = 14.9.
2. Years of life expectancy gained = 14.9 × 42 × 20% or 40% or 60%.
3. Methods of calculation and references as in Table 1.

ity reduction from screening younger women is not yet known, a similar level of benefit would seem reasonable. As for risk models, those projecting the lower levels of risk would seem more appropriate. Thus, with a 40% mortality reduction and quadratic risk projection for women age 50–59, benefits exceed risks by 62500/1 (250/0.004).

Conclusion

When compared in terms of years of life expectancy gained through early detection/years of life expectancy possibly lost from radiation, the benefits of mammographic screening appear to be considerable whereas the risk is negligible. These findings would support annual mammographic screening of all women age 40 and older.

References

Baral E, Larrson LE, Mattson B (1977) Breast cancer following irradiation of the breast. Cancer 40: 2905–2910

Boice JD, Monson RB (1977) Breast cancer following repeated fluoroscopic examinations of the chest. JNCI 59: 823–832

Committee on the Biological Effects of Ionizing Radiation (1980) The effects on populations of exposure to low levels of ionizing radiation. National Academy of Sciences Washington, DC

Feig SA (1979) Low-dose mammography, application to medical practice. JAMA 242: 2107–2109

Feig SA (1984) Radiation risk from mammography. Is it clinically significant? AJR 143: 469–475

Howe GR (1984) Epidemiology of radiogenic breast cancer. In: Boice JD Jr, Fraumeni JF Jr (eds) Radiation carcinogenesis: epidemiology and biological significance. Raven, New York, pp 119–129

Land CE, Boice JD Jr, Shore RE, et al. (1980) Breast cancer risk from low-dose exposures to ionizing radiation: results of parallel analysis of three exposed populations of women. JNCI 65: 353–376

Life Tables for the United States 1900–2050 (1983) Washington, DC: US Dept of Health and Human Services

Milbrath JR, Moskowitz M, Bauermeister D (1981) Breast cancer screening. CRC Crit Rev Diag Imaging 16: 181–218

Seidman H (1977) Screening for breast cancer in younger women: life expectancy gains and losses. An analysis according to risk indicator groups. CA 27: 66–87

Seidman H, Mushinski MH (1983) Breast cancer incidence, mortality, survival, prognosis. In: Feig SA, McLelland R (eds) Breast carcinoma: current diagnosis and treatment. Masson, New York, pp 9–46

Shapiro S, Venet W, Strax P, et al. (1982) Ten-to-fourteen-year effect of screening on breast cancer mortality. JNCI 69: 349–355

Shore RE, Hempelmann LH, Kowaluk R, et al. (1977) Breast neoplasms in women treated with x-rays for acute post-partum mastitis. JNCI 59: 813–822

Stanton L, Villafana T, Day JL, et al. (1984) Dosage evaluation in mammography. Radiology 150: 577–584

Tokunaga M, Norman JE Jr, Asano M, et al. (1979) Malignant breast neoplasms among atomic bomb survivors, Hiroshima and Nagasaki, 1950–1974. JNCI 62: 1347–1359

Tokunaga M, Land CE, Yamamota T, et al. (1984) Breast cancer among atomic bomb survivors. In: Boice JD Jr, Fraumeni JF (eds) Radiation carcinogenesis: epidemiology and biological significance. Raven, New York, pp 45–56

United Nations Scientific Committee on the Effect of Atomic Radiation (1972) Ionizing radiation: levels and effects. vol 2. United Nations, New York

Upton AC, Beebe GW, Brown JM, et al. (1977) Report of the NCI Ad Hoc Working Group on the risks associated with mammography in mass screening for the detection of breast cancer. JNCI 59: 481–493

Webster EW (1981) On the question of cancer induction by small x-ray doses. AJR 137: 647–666

Elemental Analysis of Breast Calcifications

B. M. Galkin, S. A. Feig, A. S. Patchefsky, and H. D. Muir

Departments of Radiology and Pathology, Stein Research Center, Thomas Jefferson University, 920 Chancellor Street, Philadelphia, PA 19107, USA

Introduction

For the past 37 years, ever since Leborgne (1949) demonstrated that breast cancer could be detected on the basis of radiographic images of calcifications, it has been generally accepted that all particles in the female breast are "calcifications," implying that they are chemically similar. Actually, there is no solid evidence in the literature to support this view and blind acceptance of this concept seems to have stifled inquiry about one of the most important, clinically useful markers of early breast cancer.

Several years ago it was postulated that the various sizes and shapes manifest by benign and malignant breast calcifications could result from difference in their chemical composition (Galkin et al. 1976). Techniques to test this theory have been developed (Galkin et al. 1977) and some preliminary results demonstrate the presence of different elements in some calcifications or different relative amounts of the same elements (Galkin et al. 1982; Frappart et al. 1984).

This report describes a case of breast cancer wherein the calcifications contained measurable amounts of tin.

Methods and Materials

A section of tissue about 10 cm^3 from a mastectomy specimen (histologically proven in situ and infiltrating duct carcinoma) was frozen at approximately $-20\,°C$ unfixed in a plastic container until analysis. The container was then removed from the freezer and allowed to reach room temperature. The tissue was removed to a plastic petri dish, sectioned into several smaller pieces ($<1\,cm^3$), and radiographed using a Faxitron X-ray unit and Kodak-type XTL film. Sections with calcifications were identified from the radiographs.

To digest the organic components from the tissue, several of the pieces containing calcifications were immersed in about 50 ml 5.25% sodium hypochlorite (Chlorox) for about 4 h until the gross tissue dissolved. The fluid was then filtered through a 0.2-μm-pore polycarbonate filter which was then air dried. The dry filter containing the residual inorganic material was mounted on an aluminum holder using silver adhesive and coated with gold.

The coated sample was analyzed in a scanning electron microscope (JEOL 35C) equipped with a backscattered electron detector and an X-ray energy dispersive spectrometer (Kevex 7000). The X-ray spectrum was traceable to standards of known elements. Samples of Chlorox were prepared and analyzed in a similar manner to rule out contamination from this source.

Recent Results in Cancer Research. Vol 105
© Springer-Verlag Berlin · Heidelberg 1987

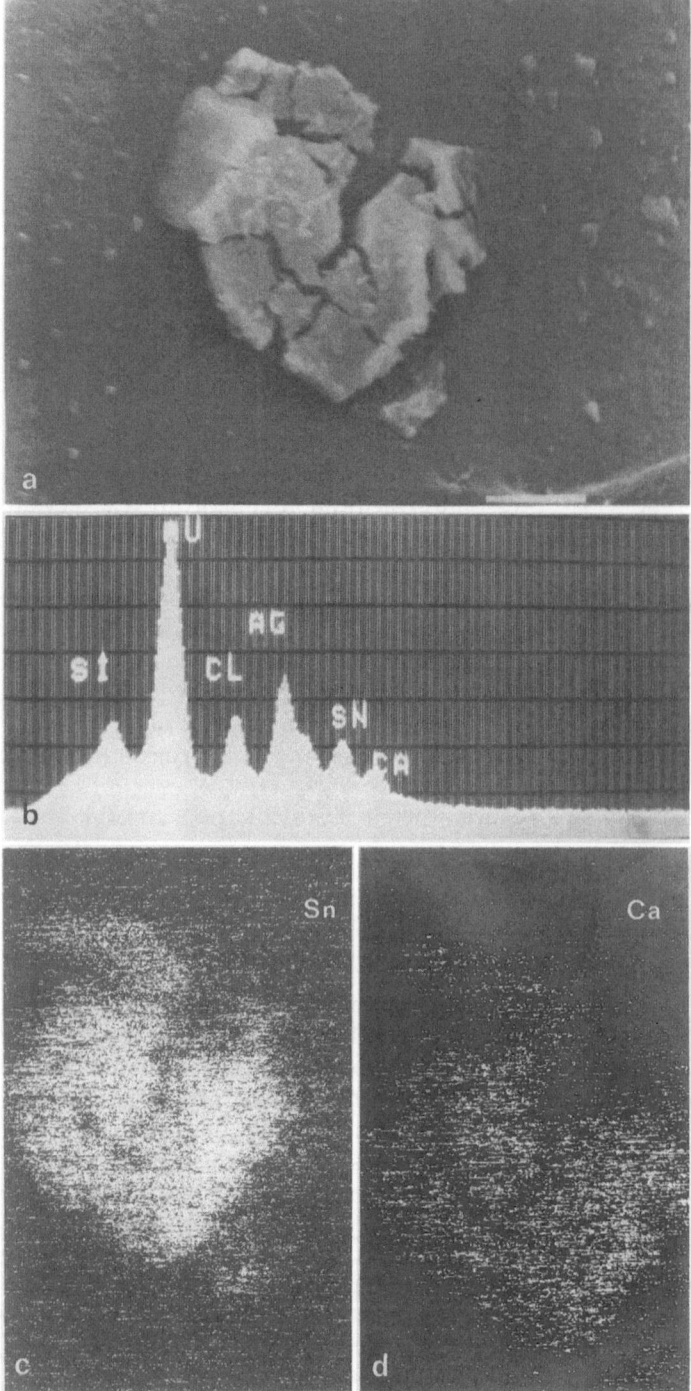

Fig. 1

Figs. 1–3 a–d. Scanning electron micrographs of breast calcifications in a tissue specimen from a histologically proven breast carcinoma. **a** Backscattered electron images; **b** X-ray spectra from the area shown in **a**; **c** characteristic X-ray maps for tin from the area shown in **a**; **d** characteristic X-ray maps for calcium from the area shown in **a**. See text for explanation of the spectra

Results

Figures 1–3 contain information for three calcifications recovered from the breast tissue. Each figure consists of (a) a backscattered electron image, (b) the X-ray spectrum from the area under view in (a), (c) an X-ray map for the element tin from the area under view in (a), and (d) an X-ray map for the element calcium from the area under view in (a). Each X-ray spectrum shows several elements; the source of each is identified as follows:

1. Silicon from the protective grease used on the window of the X-ray detector
2. Gold from the conductive coating applied to the sample
3. Chlorine from the fluid used to dissolve the tissue
4. Silver from the adhesive used to mount the sample on the specimen holder
5. Tin and calcium, presumably from the particle under view

The X-ray maps for silicon, gold, chlorine, and silver showed no preferential localization whereas the X-ray maps for tin and calcium were highly localized and clearly shaped like the particles. This validates that these three "calcifications" actually contain calcium and tin.

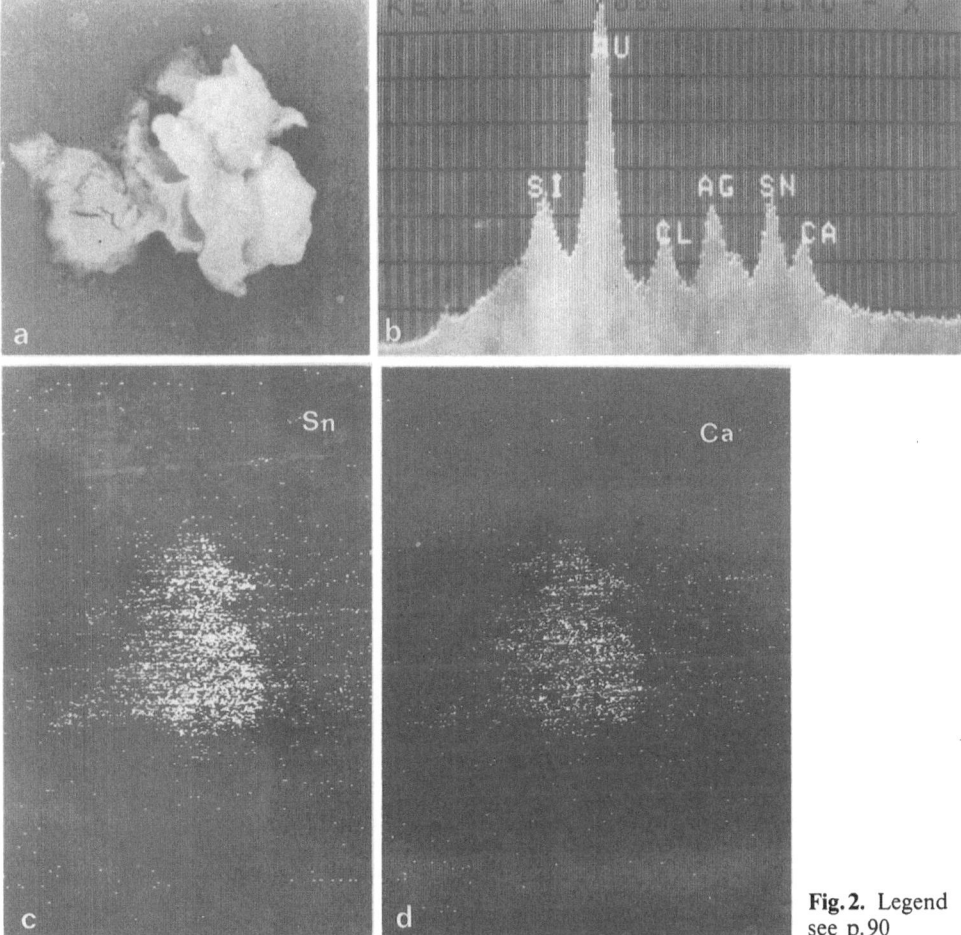

Fig. 2. Legend see p. 90

92   B. M. Galkin et al.

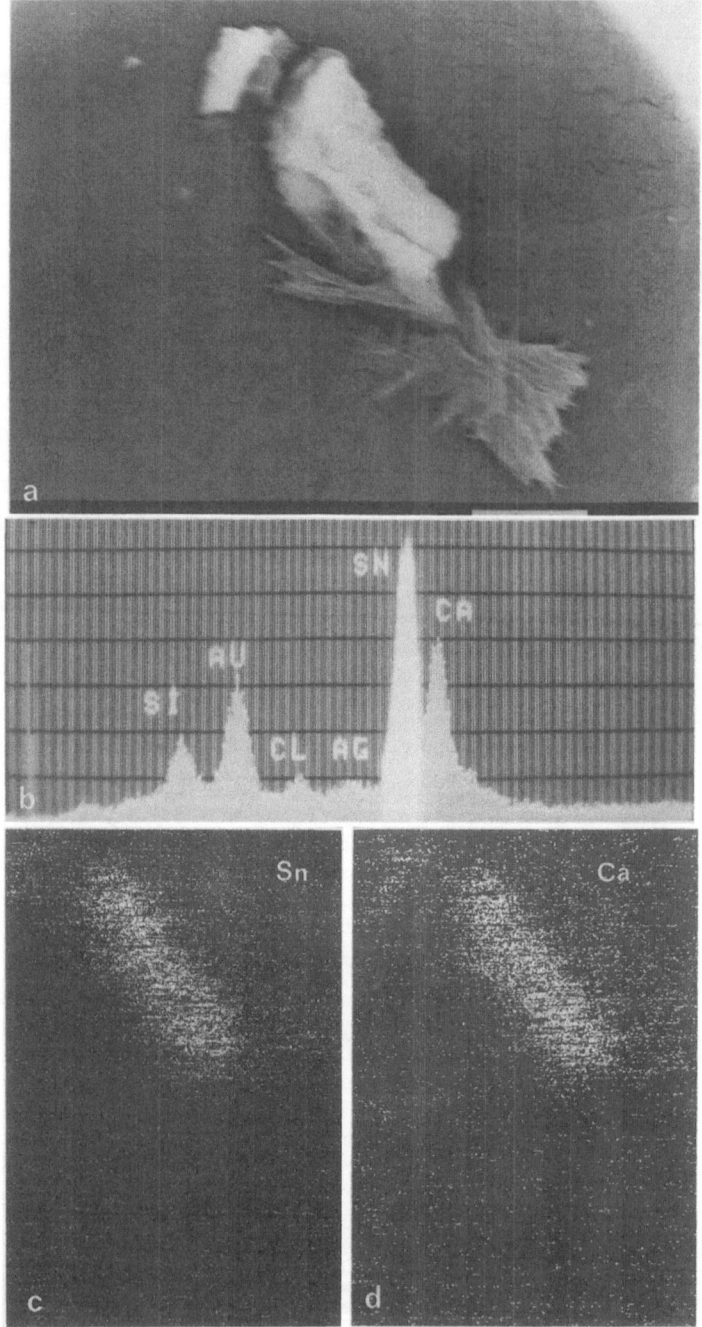

Fig. 3. Legend see p. 90

Discussion

Mammography is currently the most sensitive method for detecting breast cancer, and breast calcifications are an important radiographic marker. In many cases, analysis of the image characteristics of the calcifications may indicate to the radiologist that biopsy is either definitely indicated or contraindicated. In other instances, differentiation of benign from malignant calcifications is not certain. Unfortunately, the latter situation prevails since for every positive case of breast cancer diagnosed by mammography in the United States there are between four and eight negative biopsies performed because the radiographic signs are equivocal. While not all cases are biopsied on the sole basis of mammographic evidence of calcifications, it has been shown that over 60% of all breast cancers contain calcifications (Koehl et al. 1970).

The cost of this imprecision is enormous in terms of emotional and physical trauma for the women and anquish for their families. The financial cost is also tremendous.

It has recently been shown that a large amount of potentially useful diagnostic information can be extracted from highly magnified radiographic images of breast calcifications in excised tissue (Galkin et al. 1983). Unfortunately, much of this information cannot be obtained from state-of-the-art mammograms of the intact breast because of contrast and dose limitations (Galkin et al. 1984). This means that unless better diagnostic techniques are developed, hundreds of thousands of women will continue to be operated on unnecessarily because their benign breast conditions cannot be diagnosed any other way.

One solution to this problem would be the development of radiographic contrast agents with differential affinity for benign and malignant calcifications. Such agents would not only make the calcifications more discernable but could also provide the means for visualizing the microcalcifications associated with very early breast cancer.

There are two target populations for use of breast contrast agents. The first includes women whose mammograms are equivocal based on calcifications. Follow-up mammograms using contrast would be obtained. The calcifications would be more visible and fewer negative biopsies would result. The second population would be symptomatic young women with breasts too dense to give good mammograms. Contrast material would be used before taking the initial mammogram. Again the calcifications would be more visible and a reduction in the number of negative biopsies would result.

Previous attempts to use contrast materials for mammography have been for the most part empirical. A more rational basis for the development of such agents would be a knowledge of the chemical elements in the calcifications. The data from this report support the argument that a larger study of this type is warranted.

The results of such a study could also provide the basis for the development of contrast agents for use with other imaging modalities, e.g., computer tomography, magnetic resonance, digital radiography, and radioisotope scanning, and could also help explain the etiology of breast cancer.

Acknowledgments. We thank Ms. Patricia D. Masters for technical assistance.

Registered Trademarks. Faxitron is a registered trademark of the Hewlett-Packard Corp. XTL is a registered trademark of the Eastman Kodak Co. Chlorox is a registered trademark of the Chlorox Company.

References

Frappart L, Boudeulle M, Boumendil J, et al. (1984) Structure and composition of microcalcifications in benign and malignant lesions of the breast: study by light microscopy, transmission and scanning electron microscopy, microprobe analysis and x-ray diffraction. Hum Pathol 15: 880–889

Galkin BM, Feig SA, Patchefsky AS, et al. (1976) A new look at breast cancer calcifications. In: Digest of the fourth international conference on medical physics, Ottawa Canada Association of Physicists 25.3

Galkin BM, Feig SA, Patchefsky AS, et al. (1977) Ultrastructure and microanalysis of "benign" and "malignant" breast calcifications. Radiology 124,1: 245–249

Galkin BM, Frasca P, Feig SA, et al. (1982) Non-calcified breast particles – possible new marker of breast cancer. Invest Radiol 17,2: 119–128

Galkin BM, Feig SA, Frasca P, et al. (1983) Photomicrography of breast calcifications: correlation with histopathologic diagnosis. RadioGraphics 3,3: 450–470

Galkin BM, Feig SA, Frasca P, et al. (1984) Imaging capabilities and dose considerations of different mammographic units. Radiology 153: 365

Koehl RH, Snyder RE, Hutter RVP, et al. (1970) The incidence and significance of calcifications within operative breast specimens. Am J Clin Pathol 53: 3–53

Leborgne R (1949) Diagnostico de los tumores de la mamma por la radiografia simple. Bol Soc Cirur Uraguay 20: 407–422

Stereotaxic Fine Needle Biopsy of Nonpalpable Breast Lesions Performed by the Mammotest

G. Svane

Department of Radiology, Mammographic Section, Karolinska University Hospital, 10401 Stockholm, Sweden

Since 1976 a stereotaxic instrument for fine needle biopsy of nonpalpable breast lesions has been in use at the Department of Diagnostic Radiology, Karolinska Hospital, Stockholm, Sweden (Blomgren and Jacobsson 1977). The number of lesions examined each year has increased from 40 in 1976 to 660 in 1984. The patients are referred to this examination from different hospitals and private clinicians and private roentgenologic departments in the area of Stockholm. Only 50% are referred from our hospital.

The patient is examined lying on the examination table in a prone position with the breast to be examined hanging down through an aperture. The breast is compressed between two compression plates and two ± 15 stereoradiographs are exposed. From these the exact position of the lesion in the compressed breast can be calculated for precise insertion of the biopsy needle. After the insertion of the needle, two new stereoradiographs are exposed to check the position of the needle. The cell material sampled is smeared onto a glass slide, air dried, and handed over to the cytologist for staining and diagnosis. The screw needle biopsy instrument can be positioned with a precision of ± 1 mm. The average time of the biopsy procedure is 15 min.

A description of the Mammotest instrument, the needle biopsy technique, the technique for preoperative carbon dye marking of nonpalpable breast lesions, as well as statistical figures of the results were presented in a thesis in 1983 (Svane 1983 a, b; Nordenström et al. 1981; Svane and Silfverswärd 1983) based on case material of 527 lesions examined during the period 1976-1980. From June 1980 to December 1982 1026 lesions were stereotaxically examined; 214 were surgically excised (Table 1-3).

Table 1. Roentgenologic, cytologic, and histopathologic evaluation

Roentgenology	Cytology		Histology	
Probably benign 119 lesions	Benign	96	Benign	91
			Cancer	5
	Probably cancer	3	Benign	2
			Cancer	1
	Cancer	20	Benign	–
			Cancer	20
Probably cancer or cancer 95 lesions	Benign	18	Benign	6
			Cancer	12
	Probably cancer	5	Benign	–
			Cancer	5
	Cancer	72	Benign	3
			Cancer	69

Table 2. Cytologic evaluation in relation to histopathologic evaluation

Cytology	Histology	
	Benign	Cancer
Benign	97	17
Probably cancer	2	6
Cancer	3	89

Table 3. Size in mammograms of malignant tumor within various cytologic groups

Cytology	Tumor diameter (mm)				
	⩽5	6–10	11–15	16–20	⩾21
Benign (17)	4	9	2	1	1
Probably cancer (6)	–	4	1	1	–
Cancer (89)	12	44	15	9	9

The smears were examined at the Department of Cytology, Karolinska Hospital, and finally rescrutinized by Prof. Sixten Franzén. The histopathologic diagnosis was performed at different hospitals and rescrutinized by Assistant Prof. Lambert Skoog. The mammograms were rescrutinized by myself.

Fifteen percent of the patients referred for stereotaxic needle biopsy were referred for preoperative carbon marking of the lesion at the same time. The position of the lesion is determined by stereoradiographs. A water suspension of carbon is injected through the stereographically positioned needle from the lesion out to the skin while the needle is withdrawn. The needle track is thereby stained black by carbon.

References

Blomgren J, Jacobsson B, Nordenström B (1977) Stereotaxic instrument for needle biopsy of the mamma. Am J Roentgenol 129: 121

Nordenström B, Rydén H, Svane G (1981) Breast. In Zornoza J (ed) Percutaneous needle biopsy. Williams and Wilkins, Baltimore p 43

Svane G (1983a) Stereotaxic needle biopsy of non-palpable breast lesions. Doctoral Thesis, Karolinska Institute, Stockholm

Svane G (1983b) A stereotaxic technique for preoperative marking of non-palpable breast lesions. Acta Radiol Diagn 24: 145

Svane G, Silfverswärd C (1983) Stereotaxic needle biopsy of non-palpable breast lesions. Acta Radiol Diagn 24: 283

Changing Aspects of Biopsy of the Breast: Is Breast Biopsy a Prognostic Hazard?

S. Watt-Boolsen, M. Blichert-Toft, J. A. Andersen, and K. West Andersen

Surgical Department, Division of Endocrine Surgery, and Institute of Pathology,
Odense University Hospital, 5000 Odense C, Denmark

Introduction

The attitude concerning breast biopsy in patients with malignant or suspected malignant mammary lesions has varied since biopsy was first carried out in the middle of the nineteenth century (McGraw and Hartman 1933). Initially, the main disagreement was about the overall necessity for breast biopsy. Later, the issues were when and how to do the biopsy. Today, most surgeons probably agree that ablative mammary procedures should not be undertaken unless malignancy has been verified by microscopic examinations of the suspected lesions. This almost universal agreement concerning the necessity for microscopic examination may in part be due to the recognition of the inaccuracy of the clinical examination in early malignancies of the breast. With the introduction of subclinical cancer, the microscopic examination has become indispensable.

A major topic has been, and still is, whether or not the biopsy procedure in itself has deleterious effects on the course of the disease. An incisional biopsy or even a needle biopsy may theoretically promote tumor cell spread locally or distantly via opened blood and lymph vessels. However, by doing a complete removal of the tumor for biopsy purposes this problem may be solved. Consequently, wide excisional biopsy was strongly recommended by some surgeons (Adair 1933; Harrington 1933; Harrington 1935; Storrs 1952; Shallow et al. 1953; Urban 1978), whereas others, especially Haagensen (Haagensen and Stout 1951; Haagensen 1971), virtually considered excisional biopsy impossible except in very minute lesions. He claimed that "the carcinoma frequently infiltrates far beyond the grossly visible limits of the disease, and no surgeon can hope that a local excision will get beyond it."

Therefore, Haagensen advocated a small incisional biopsy for frozen section, followed by immediate radical operation, if malignancy was proved. In minute lesions, a total removal was aimed at during biopsy.

Before considering the potential hazards of breast biopsy in detail, various biopsy procedures and related pathoanatomical procedures will be dealt with.

Biopsy Methods

One way of performing a breast biopsy is by using an open biopsy, the so-called knife biopsy. Another method is closed biopsy, the so-called needle biopsy.

Knife biopsy may be excisional or incisional, the former indicating total tumor removal and the latter removal of only a small wedge of the tumor. Needle biopsy comprises the use of either a core-cutting needle or a fine-needle, mounted on a syringe for aspiration of detached cells. Biopsy with a knife and with a core-cutting needle provides tissue for histological examination as opposed to fine needle aspiration, by which only a sample for cytological examination is provided.

In open biopsy, the predictive value of a positive (PV_{pos}) or negative (PV_{neg}) histological finding in paraffin-embedded blocks is 1.0, if the biopsy is representative and the pathologist is experienced in breast pathology. In needle biopsy, representativity is a major problem, since the needle may miss the tumor. However, with increased experience the failure rate diminishes (Dixon et al. 1984).

Core-cutting needle biopsy performed by employing a pistol grip has been demonstrated to have a PV_{pos} of 1.0 (95% confidence limits, 0.84–1.0) and PV_{neg} of 1.0 (95% confidence limits, 0.66–1.0) in palpable tumors suspeted to be malignant of 1.5 cm or more in diameter (Nielsen et al. 1983). The biopsy can usually be used for frozen sections with a similar degree of reliability.

Fine needle aspiration biopsy for cytological evaluation has been found to have a PV_{pos} ranging from 0.90 to 0.98 and a PV_{neg} of from 0.97 to 1.0 (Olsen et al. 1978; Shabot et al. 1982; Dixon et al. 1984; Hermansen et al. 1984). The reliability, however, is very dependent upon technical experience (Dixon et al. 1984) and upon cytological expertise. One disadvantage is that differentiation between invasive and noninvasive cancer is not possible by the use of cytology.

The decision of which biopsy method to employ mainly depends upon the purpose of the biopsy and the type of breast lesion. In our opinion, the purpose of breast biopsy is to achieve a definitive diagnosis, i. e., to establish whether or not the lesion is malignant, and in the case of malignancy, whether the adenocarcinoma is invasive or noninvasive. With that background, we prefer histological diagnosis by using knife biopsy or core-cutting needle biopsy.

Our current policy regarding pathoanatomical procedures in the case of open biopsy is to forward the unfixed biopsy specimen immediatly to the pathologist. The tissue specimen is then cut into 2-mm-thin slices which are assessed macroscopically for areas suspected of malignancy. Frozen sections are examined only if such areas are found. If no gross lesions suspected of malignancy are detected, the whole specimen is fixed, embedded in paraffin, cut, and stained with hematoxylin-eosin for further examination.

If the mammographic examination has revealed microcalcifications, tissue specimens or paraffin blocks are X-rayed to look for suspicious areas for a more detailed histological examination.

As to core-cutting needle biopsy, this method is reserved for solid palpable tumors suspected of malignancy and with a diameter of 1.5 cm or more. If malignancy is verified, definitive surgery is carried out; if not, the tumor is excised for further examination.

Previous Studies on Excisional Versus Incisional Biopsy

Adair (1933), dealing with the subject of breast biopsy, wrote "It must be stated in all scientific fairness that there seems to be much of theory but little of scientific proof of the dire results of the different methods of biopsy." This statement still holds in the sense that undeniable proof of the deleterious effects of breast biopsy has not been provided. The necessary randomized study has never been performed. However, three reports may be interpreted as stating that there is a damaging effect of incisional breast biopsy compared with excisional biopsy.

Pierce et al. (1956) investigated the 5-year survival rate in 55 patients who had undergone excisional biopsy before delayed radical operation, and similar criteria in another 41 patients who had had incisional biopsy also previous to delayed radical operation. The survival rates were 70.9% and 47.5%, respectively. However, the results were not analyzed with respect to disease stage.

Hattori et al. (1980) reported on the basis of a retrospective questionare investigation comprising one-third of the membership institutions of the Japan Mammary Cancer Society which found that patients with T_1, T_2, and T_{3+4} tumors had a significantly superior prognosis, when excisional biopsy had been attempted, compared with those with incisional biopsy. The 5-year recurrence rates in T_1 patients with incisional/excisional biopsy were 14.5%/9.5%, in T_2 patients 25.9%/18.3%, and in T_{3+4} patients 54.5%/34.8%. This part of their investigation comprised 4694 patients, who had had either immediate or delayed radical mastectomy. The results were not analyzed with respect to nodal stage. Furthermore, the data reported strongly suggest that only in approximately two-thirds of the patients in whom excisional biopsy had been attempted had this in fact been carried out, as indicated by the absense of residual foci of cancer in the resected specimen.

Andersen et al. (1984) studied 3-year cumulative recurrence-free survival rates (RFS) in 3264 patients who had had frozen sections taken followed immediately by total mastectomy and partial axillary dissection. These patients comprised a part of a group of Danish breast cancer patients who were included in a prospective nationwide study done by the Danish Breast Cancer Cooperative Group (DBCG). According to the protocol, excisional biopsy was aimed at. Andersen et al. (1984) compared RFS in patients with or without residual cancer tissue (RCT) in the mastectomy specimen. In high-risk patients, the rate of recurrence was significantly higher when RCT was present. In the premenopausal group with or without RCT, RFS was 55% and 81%, respectively. Correspondingly, in the postmenopausal group the values were 60% and 70%, respectively. Differences in RFS in subsets of patients with or without RCT were not related to tumor size, anaplasia grading, number of metastatic lymph nodes, or several other histopathological characteristics. Also in low-risk patients, the presence of RCT was associated with a higher recurrence rate, albeit not significantly.

Although neither of these studies was randomized with respect to excisional or incisional biopsy, the results indicate a potentially dire effect of incisional biopsy.

Present Study of Excisional Versus Incisional Biopsy

The observations reported by Andersen et al. (1984) above have been reevaluated after an additional observation time of 4 years, completing a 7-year follow-up period.

Patients and Methods

The present series comprises 3975 patients. They all fulfilled the criteria for entering the DBCG-77 protocols dealing with operable breast cancer. The study design appears in Fig. 1. Low-risk patients comprised those with a tumor of 5 cm or less in diameter, no histologically demonstrable invasion to skin or deep fascia, and no metastatic axillary lymph nodes. High-risk patients were those with a tumor of 5 cm or more in diameter and/or histologically demonstrable invasion to skin or deep fascia and/or spread to axillary lymph nodes. No patient had any sign of metastatic spread, based on physical examination, chest

LOW-RISK GROUP
Premenopausal and postmenopausal patients:

Surgery ⟶ Watch policy

HIGH-RISK GROUP
Premenopausal patients:

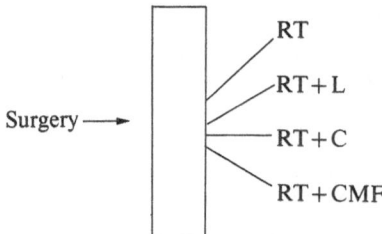

Postmenopausal patients:

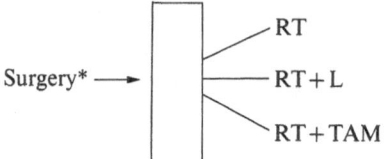

Fig. 1. Study design in the DBCG-77 trials.
*Surgery, total mastectomy + partial axillary
dissection; *RT*, postoperative radiotherapy;
L, levamisole; *C*, cyclophosphamide;
CmF, C + methotrexate + 5-fluorouracil;
TAM, tamoxifen

X-ray, and bone scintigraphy. They all underwent open biopsy and frozen section, immediately followed by total mastectomy and partial axillary dissection in one stage.

Residual cancer tissue (RCT) was defined by the presence of cancer left in the biopsy
cavity wall in the mastectomy specimen. Routine pathological procedures comprised
macroscopic investigation of the wall of the biopsy cavity and microscopic investigation
of two or more paraffin-embedded tissue sections.

Recurrence was defined as the first locoregional recurrence and/or distant metastasis
discovered during regular follow-up, comprising clinical examination and chest X-ray.
Deaths, irrespective of cause, were calculated as recurrences.

The cumulative recurrence-free survival rates were compared by the log-rank test. A P
value less of than. 0.05 was considered significant.

Results

The low-risk group comprised 1972 patients, of whom 673 were premenopausal and
1299 postmenopausal. The high-risk group comprised 2003 patients, of whom 741 were
premenopausal and 1262 postmenopausal.

Residual cancer tissue was found in 33% of low-risk patients and in 62% of high-risk
patients. Both within the low-risk and the high-risk group, RCT occurred with the same
frequency in pre- and postmenopausal patients.

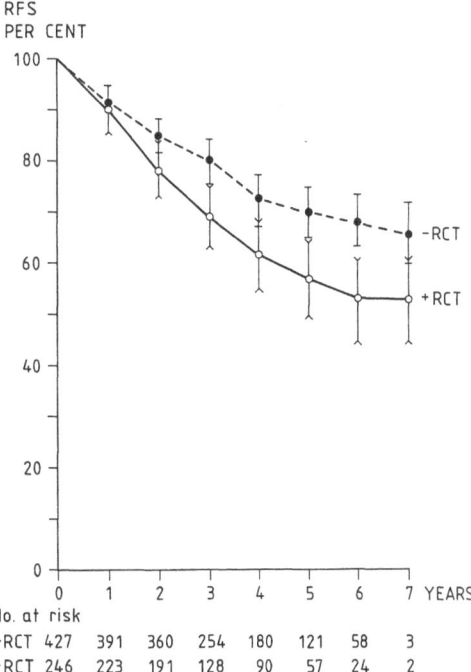

RFS
PER CENT

Fig. 2. Recurrence-free survival *(RFS)* for low-risk premenopausal patients with primary breast carcinoma with *(+ RCT)* or without residual cancer tissue *(– RCT)* in the mastectomy specimen. The 95% confidence limits are indicated

No. at risk

	0	1	2	3	4	5	6	7
–RCT	427	391	360	254	180	121	58	3
+RCT	246	223	191	128	90	57	24	2

Recurrence was observed in 507 low-risk patients and in 676 high-risk patients. In low-risk patients, the ratio between locoregional and distant metastasis was 1:1. In high-risk patients this ratio was 1:3.

The cumulative recurrence-free survival rates (RFS) in patients with or without RCT are given in Fig. 2–5. The number of patients at risk and the 95% confidence limits based on Greenwood's estimate are also indicated.

It appears that the presence of RCT is associated with a significantly higher recurrence risk in all groups. Thus, low-risk, premenopausal patients (Fig. 2) with or without RCT showed an RFS after 7 years of 53% and 66%, respectively (log-rank 8.8, $P<0.003$). In low-risk, postmenopausal patients (Fig. 3) with or without RCT, the RFS after 7 years was 55% and 62%, respectively (log-rank 7.7, $P<0.006$). High-risk, premenopausal patients (Fig. 4) with or without RCT showed an RFS after 7 years of 49% and 70%, respectively (log-rank 30.5, $P<0.0001$). In the high-risk, postmenopausal patients (Fig. 5) with or without RCT, RFS after 7 years was 35% and 58%, respectively (log-rank 31.5, $P<0.0001$).

In high-risk patients, the association between the presence of RCT and higher recurrence rate is distinct already within the 1st year of observation. On the other hand, it is not until after approximately 5 years of observation that this becomes clearly visible in the low-risk group.

Discussion

The finding that RCT is associated with significantly increased recurrence rate not only in high-risk, but also in low-risk, patients poses important questions. Firstly, what is the prognostic power of RCT alone and in combination with traditionally recognized prog-

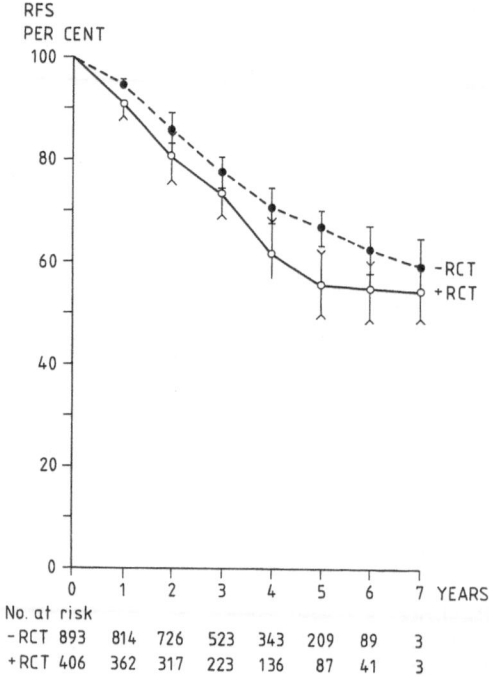

No. at risk

	0	1	2	3	4	5	6	7
-RCT	893	814	726	523	343	209	89	3
+RCT	406	362	317	223	136	87	41	3

Fig. 3. Recurrence-free survival *(RFS)* for low-risk postmenopausal patients with primary breast carcinoma with *(+ RCT)* or without residual cancer tissue *(− RCT)* in the mastectomy specimen. The 95% confidence limits are indicated

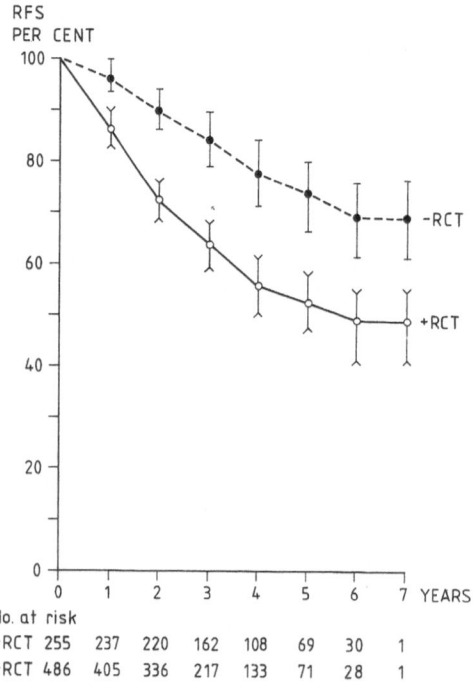

No. at risk

	0	1	2	3	4	5	6	7
-RCT	255	237	220	162	108	69	30	1
+RCT	486	405	336	217	133	71	28	1

Fig. 4. Recurrence-free survival *(RFS)* for high-risk premenopausal patients with primary breast carcinoma with *(+ RCT)* or without residual cancer tissue *(− RCT)* in the mastectomy specimen. The 95% confidence limits are indicated

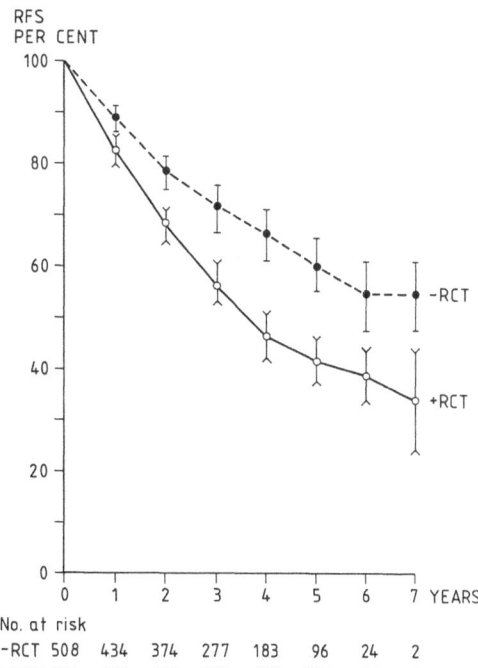

Fig. 5. Recurrence-free survival *(RFS)* for high-risk postmenopausal patients with primary breast carcinoma with *(+ RCT)* or without residual cancer tissue *(− RCT)* in the mastectomy specimen. The 95% confidence limits are indicated

nostic criteria such as nodal status, tumor size, and anaplasia grading? Secondly, is the relationship between RCT and increased recurrence causal or does it merely reflect differences in tumor biology?

The prognostic power of RCT alone appears in Fig. 2–5, where the 95% confidence limits for each observation of RFS are indicated. The prognostic power of RCT in combination with other, strong prognostic criteria is under investigation at present. However, the study by Andersen et al. (1984) and our preliminary results indicate that RCT is an independent prognostic factor.

The very important question of a causal relationship between incisional biopsy and increased rate of recurrence cannot be definitively answered. Although the DBCG-77 study was prospective, the patients were not randomized to either excisional or incisional biopsy. Excisional biopsy was advocated in the protocols. The data do not allow us to establish whether or not excisional biopsy was attempted. Therefore, a failure rate cannot be established. However, we have no sound cause for believing that the ratio planned excisional/planned incisional biopsy differs among the protocols. It can therefore be argued that the major part of the patients are self-randomized to excisional or incisional biopsy, the latter indicated by the presence of RCT in the mastectomy specimen. Our findings must be weighed against this background. Moreover, conduction of a prospective randomized study would probably be considered unethical, due to the potential hazard of incisional biopsy. Furthermore, one would have to solve the problem that attempted excisional biopsy may fail. According to Hattori et al. (1980), approximately one-third of attempted excisional biopsies will in fact be incisional.

Although the DBCG-77 study design does not allow definitive conclusions as to causality, the results indicate a potential hazard of incisional biopsy. However, certain factors disfavor a causal relationship. Firstly, causality would require the existence of ultrarapidacting tumor growth- or spread-promoting mechanisms, since the breast was removed within a very short time after biopsy. Such mechanisms have been suggested, but have never been undeniably documented (Moore 1867, Tyzzer 1913). Secondly, one-stage mastectomy should result in a better prognosis than delayed mastectomy, if cutting through tumor tissue resulted in production of tumor-promoting factors. The superiority of one-stage mastectomy has not been documented (Abramson 1976, Fisher 1984, Bertario et al. 1985). Thirdly, radical operations should result in reduced cancer mortality compared with less radical procedures. That this is not the case is a well-known fact. Fourthly, if the explanation is causal and not biological, RCT should be present in approximately the same percentage in low-risk and high-risk patients. In our study, RCT occurred in only one-third of low-risk patients, but in two-thirds of high-risk patients. Fifthly, but of utmost importance, the difference in RFS should appear at the same time in high- and low-risk patients, if the association between incisional biopsy and lower RFS was to be causal. However, in high-risk patients, the difference was evident already after 1 year of observation, but not until 5 years of observation in low-risk patients. Thus, it is more likely that our findings reflect tumor biology rather than causality.

Nevertheless, since causality cannot be undeniably ruled out, we find that open biopsy should preferably be excisional. Whether the prognostic significance of RCT adds significantly to the already known powerful prognostic criteria in breast cancer is under investigation.

Whether or not increased risk of recurrence is associated with other forms of biopsy, e. g., needle biopsy, remains to be established. In our prospective DBCG-82 protocols, this subject is dealt with.

Acknowledgment. The study has been supported by a grant from Consul General Oscar Zimmermann's Fund.

References

Abramson DJ (1976) Delayed mastectomy after outpatient breast biopsy. Long-term survival study. Am J Surg 132: 596–598

Adair FE (1933) Clinical manifestations of early cancer of the breast. N Engl J Med 208: 1250–1255

Andersen JA, Blichert-Toft M, Kjærgård J et al. (1984) Prognostic significance of residual cancer tissue after diagnostic biopsy in breast carcinoma. Three year short-term results. Eur J Cancer Clin Oncol 20: 765–770

Bertario L, Reduzzi D, Piromalli D et al. (1985) Outpatient biopsy of breast cancer. Ann Surg 201: 64–67

Dixon JM, Anderson TJ, Lamb J et al. (1984) Fine needle aspiration cytology, in relationships to clinical examination and mammography in the diagnosis of a solid breast mass. Br J Surg 71: 593–596

Fisher ER (1984) The impact of pathology on the biologic, diagnostic, prognostic and therapeutic considerations in breast cancer. Surg Clin North Am 64: 1073–1093

Haagensen CD, Stout AP (1951) Carcinoma of the breast. Ann Surg 134: 151–172

Haagensen CD (1971) Diseases of the breast, 2nd edn. Saunders, Philadelphia, pp 143–145

Harrington SW (1933) Carcinoma of the breast: surgical treatment and results five, ten and fifteen years after radical amputation. Surg Gynecol Obstet 56: 438–441

Harrington SW (1935) Unilateral cancer of the breast treated by surgical operation and radiation. Surg Gynecol Obstet 60: 499–504

Hattori T, Niimoto M, Nakano A et al. (1980) Biopsy of the breast. Jpn J Surg 10: 270–276

Hermansen C, Poulsen HS, Jensen J et al. (1984) Palpable breast tumors: "triple diagnosis" and operative strategy. Acta Chir Scand 150: 625–628

McGraw AB, Hartman FW (1933) Present status of the biopsy. JAMA 101: 1205–1209

Moore CH (1867) On the influence of inadequate operations on the theory of breast cancer. R Chir Soc 1: 244–280

Nielsen HO, Blichert-Toft M, Hariri J (1983) The pistomat needle biopsy for preoperative diagnosis of breast tumors. Ugeskr Laeger 145: 234–236

Olsen TS, Egedorf J, Ibsen J et al. (1978) Employment of fine-needle aspiration cytology in the diagnosis and therapy of tumors of the breast. Ugeskr Laeger 140: 2973–2975

Pierce EH, Clagett OT, McDonald JR et al. (1956) Biopsy of the breast followed by delayed radical mastectomy. Surg Gynecol Obstet 103: 559–564

Shabot MM, Goldberg IM, Schick P et al. (1982) Aspiration cytology is superior to Tru-cut needle biopsy in establishing the diagnosis of clinically suspicious breast masses. Ann Surg 196: 122–126

Shallow TA, Wagner FB, Colcher RE (1953) Adequate breast biopsy. Arch Surg 67: 526–536

Storrs HG (1952) The role of excision biopsy in lesions of the breast. Am Surg 18: 1199–1206

Tyzzer EE (1913) Factors in the production and growth of tumor metastasis. J Med Res 28: 309–333

Urban JA (1978) Management of operable breast cancer: the surgeons view. Cancer 42: 2066–2077

Self-Examination in Early Detection of Breast Cancer: Is It Effective?

G. Gästrin

Ståhlbergsvägen 6F55, 00570 Helsingfors 57, Finland

It is well known that in more than 90% of all breast cancer cases, the women have – as a first step – discovered symptoms or signs of breast cancer themselves, and then sooner or later referred themselves to a physician. Such quite accidental touching or looking at one's breasts is sometimes referred to as some sort of breast self-examination (BSE). Under these circumstances the answer to the question in the title must be: "No," BSE is not effective.

However, the answer is "Yes" when speaking seriously about the capability of a woman to learn to know her own breasts while they are healthy and her capability to recognize changes from what is normal for her and additionally her activity when referring herself to mammography examination immediately if changes from normal occur.

The accidental discovery of a symptom leads to the detection of breast cancer tumors that are 2 cm in diameter or more, but a systematic BSE month after month discovers symptoms of tumours that are 0.5–1 cm in diameter only.

Because of a regrettable lack of distinction between the nature of BSE as such in more or less accidental approaches, on one hand, and more comprehensive BSE-containing program approaches on the other hand, comparisons have been made by some authors between the clinical effect of BSE and the effect of mammography examination. This comparison is not relevant because the latter is a means of clinical diagnosis, while BSE as such is only a woman's search for self-detectable symptoms by inspection and palpation.

Other authors have compared the effect of BSE as such with mammography screening. This is irrelevant as well, because the latter constitutes an organizational system within society, while BSE as such is not. This paper discusses the three different BSE approaches and also the role of BSE when used as part of a comprehensive, BSE-containing program.

BSE as such is only a temporary activity by a woman, who has in one way or another been motivated to inspect and palpate her breasts. The performance of BSE is not automatically integrated in any wider context and it includes no referral system in the case of occurrence of breast cancer symptoms. Certain knowledge, disseminated by the mass media, about the need for BSE causes uncertainty, fear, and pessimism.

BSE-containing programs of the traditional type constitute the teaching of the BSE technique. The combination of such a teaching procedure with, e. g., the Papanicolaou test raises problems because of the much too long intervals between the screening procedures.

A comprehensive and continuous program including BSE implies the transfer of partial responsibility to women themselves in line with the current approach of establishing interrelations between healthy populations and health-care services. The Finnish Mama program consists of (a) an initial teaching procedure, (b) a surveillance system with the use of personal calendars during the continuous program, and (c) a self-referral system to prompt mammography examination if symptoms of breast cancer are detected by the women themselves.

This comprehensive BSE-containing program has been referred to by experts of the WHO Cancer Unit in Geneva as a new sort of screening test.

When speaking about screening tests for the early detection of breast cancer, the two organizational systems conventional mammography screening and Mama program screening could be discussed and compared. In conventional screening for breast cancer, where mammography examination constitutes the screening test, symptom-free women are examined at certain intervals. Tumors 0.1 cm in diameter are detected, but because of the high cost only limited groups of women in the world can be involved.

In Mama program screening the test is not a single procedure at a given date, but constitutes a continuous, multicomponent program containing BSE on a monthly basis year after year. Women in the program are able to detect tumors 1 cm in diameter and the program can be applied in large populations in developed and developing countries without requiring a substantial increase in health resources, provided there is a health care system with adequate diagnosis and treatment resources.

The fundamentals of the Mama program are:

- The capability of a woman to learn to know her breasts while they are symptomfree and to identify changes from what is normal for her
- Person to person communication together with certain surveillance influences health behavior (regular BSE and self-referral to mammography examination, if needed on the basis of self-detection of breast cancer symptoms), while one-way communication with leaflets or lectures on the BSE technique mainly influences knowledge, but not health behavior
- Public health care systems in developed and partly in developing countries today have the capacity to take care of persons who show up because of self-detected symptoms of a disease.

The three main features of the comprehensive, continuous Mama program are:

1. Initial communication of the key message is performed face to face. The message is aimed at motivating women to achieve a certain health behavior concerning (a) monthly breast self-examination and (b) prompt self-referral to mammography examination (or an intermediate physician) if changes from normal occur in the breasts. The message contains information on the normal breast pattern at different ages, self-detectable nonmalignant and malignant changes, the cautious BSE technique, the need for monthly BSE, and explanations about the different steps of the Mama program entity in practice in the area in question.
2. A continuous surveillance system is established with personal "calendars" to be filled in and annually renewed. Each woman having attended the initial information session will receive a calendar with the following purposes: (1) to remind the woman of the BSE technique and the necessity to practice it regularly once a month, (2) to facilitate registration of any changes in the breasts detected during BSE, (3) to provide information on how to act when abnormalities are detected including the name of the physician to be consulted first, and (4) to serve as a means of feedback.
3. There is a self-referral system to mammography examination in case changes from normal are detected. The health personnel in charge of the program make advance arrangements with mammography unit members in the area in question. The address is entered into the calendar of each woman. This is aimed at avoiding delay for the patients and doctors.

The Mama program has been tested in a population study in Finland in 1972-1975. The aims of the study were:

- To determine the magnitude of the effect of a comprehensive BSE-containing program on breast cancer detection rate and stage, and on reduction in mortality from breast cancer following earlier detection of the disease.
- To explore whether a comprehensive breast self-examination-containing program can be considered an integral part of the public health care approach aimed at controlling the problem of breast cancer.
- To determine the behavioural, cultural, and psychological problems which can occur when well women are invited to participate in a breast cancer early detection program, with a BSE-containing comprehensive program as the screening component
- To provide the data for estimation of the cost and resource needs of a comprehensive program for early breast cancer detection. In the Finnish population study there were 56000 women enrolled, one physician and one nurse who gave the key message, and 20 radiologists, who carried out the mammography examinations.

Conclusions about the results are drawn on the basis of comparisons with psychological and behavioural findings prior to intervention and clinical findings according to the figures of the Finnish Cancer Registry during the year before the intervention started. Mortality figures are compared with data from the period 1966-1970 registered by the Finnish Cancer Registry. The results are published in the book *Breast Cancer Control - An Early Detection Programme* (Gästrin 1981). The result of such a comprehensive program will depend on how far women can be persuaded to practice breast self-examination on a regular basis and to show up, as agreed, if changes from normal are detected by inspection or palpation.

Among the psychosocial and behavioural findings the following can be mentioned:

- Monthly BSE performance rate increased from only 1% to 68% in the group of women who received the initial information in groups and a personal calendar for monthly notes. Similar results are shown in later studies in Sweden.
- Two percent of the women in the intervention group showed up with self-detected breast cancer symptoms. According to returned questionnaires the interest to start the program was raised by the trustworthy initial information by a medically trained key person, and the interest in going on with the program was achieved by factors associated with keeping calendar notes.

The work load on mammography radiologists was minimal. Out of 56000 women in the project, 750 showed up at those 20 radiologists' consultations, which fits well into the public health care approach in most countries.

The detection rate of new breast cancer cases was 90 cases in the group of 56000 women (51 expected according to the compared age groups). The program discovered three times more cases in women below 50 years of age than in the comparison group.

The detected new cases were, on average, less advanced than in the compared population, which had accidentally discovered symptoms. Seventy percent of the cases were local to the breast (compared with 48% in the population). There was a greater than usual proportion of in situ carcinoma cases: 4.4% (control population, 2.4%).

As far as mortality from breast cancer in the project group women is concerned, there are some data available from a 5 year follow-up. Among the women who had their breast cancer detected during the 1st year of the Mama program (90 cases) 28 died (31%), which is a reduction of 31% compared to the mortality during the period 1966-1970 (45%).

Among the new breast cancer cases detected during the second project year (35 cases) 9 died (26%), which is a reduction of 42% compared to the mortality during the period 1966–1970. The mortality from breast cancer in a 10 years follow-up will be published later.

Cost per new detected case was about $ 200 US.

In Finland the National Board of Health gave information letters about the implementation of the Mama program on a national basis to public health centers for the first time in 1975 and they have been repeated. Since 1975 nearly 1 million women have in one way or another been enrolled in the continuous Mama program through channels of public health care and occupational health care. Since 1975 it has been shown that crude incidence rates of new detected breast cancer increased sharply and more than predicted by the Finnish Cancer Registry for the period 1973–1980.

Carrying out the Mama program at a national level requires certain initiatives, continuous activities, and certain working aids. The following steps are needed:

- Identification of adequate environments. Decision makers within public health care and occupational health care should decide about the introduction of the comprehensive program. The target could be all women over 30 years of age. In many developed countries about 70% of these women can be reached by occupational health care facilities.
- Cooperation with mammography unit members has to be established in order to take care of those women who show up with self-detected symptoms (about 2% of the Mama program participants per year).
- Nomination of appropriate key persons. Among medical and paramedical personnel a key person needs to be nominated and the work with the Mama program should be an integral part of her/his daily routine.
- Assistance of the key persons in their everyday work. "Teaching kits" have already been published which are developed and tested during the Finnish trial as well as in Sweden and the WHO project in Leningrad and Moscow. They contain: the methodological description of the program, the initial message to the program participants, a demonstration wall chart, overhead pictures, and the calendars for 1 years use to be renewed on an annual basis.

When implementing the comprehensive, continuous BSE-containing Mama program at a local or national level, certain baseline data are required that are available from the experiences in Finland. Extrapolations have been made for different cultural and social environments in developed and developing countries, and have been published in the book *Breast Cancer Control* (Gästrin 1981). After publication of this book, the WHO Cancer Unit in Geneva discussed the use of the Mama program especially for areas where mammography screening and physical examination of the breasts are not practicable as public health policies. The Mama program was discussed at the WHO International Meeting for Formulation of Preventive Strategies in Cancer 1981. It was considered in greater detail by a group of experts convened by WHO in 1983. It was agreed to further test the efficacy of the continuous BSE-containing program as a potential means of reduction in mortality from breast cancer in a population of 186000 women aged 40–64 years, randomized for study and control groups in Moscow and Leningrad in cooperation with the Petrov Research Institute in Leningrad.

As a replication of the Finnish Mama study, the actual education is based on person to person communication using the Finnish message and printed material. The feedback information is received from calendars as in the Finnish program and there is a self-referral system with intermediate physicians. The study is expected to result in the accrual of more than 700 new breast cancer cases of which 380 will be cumulative deaths. The study is expected to be powerful enough to come to a conclusive judgment on the value of the comprehensive and continuous Mama program in the society of the USSR, assuming that at least 67% of women in the study group practiced breast self-examination on a regular basis, as did the women in the Finnish study.

References

Gästrin G (1981) Breast cancer control – an early detection programme. Almqvist and Wiksell International, Uppsala Sweden

Gästrin G (1986) Självundersökning av brösten – Mamametoden. Teaching kit including manual, over-head pictures, wall chart and calendars. Folkhälsan-Kansanterveys, Helsingfors Finland

Evaluation of Breast Microcalcifications by Means of Optically Magnified Tissue Specimen Radiographs

S. A. Feig, B. M. Galkin, and H. D. Muir

Department of Radiology, Stein Research Center, Thomas Jefferson University Hospital, 920 Chancellor Street, Philadelphia, PA 19107, USA

Although the presence of microcalcifications in a breast cancer mass seen on mammography was first reported by Salomon (1913), Leborgne (1949) was the first to recognize that microcalcifications can represent the only mammographic manifestation of carcinoma. Since then, it has become apparent that 29%–48% of nonpalpable carcinomas are visible on the basis of microcalcifications alone (Table 1).

Microcalcifications are especially important as a sign of early breast cancer. Moskowitz (1983) found that 71% (29/41) of nonpalpable minimal cancers (noninfiltrating cancers and cancers smaller than 0.5 cm) were detected on the basis of microcalcifications alone. In another study, Feig (1977) found that 89% (56/63) of nonpalpable in situ ductal carcinomas were seen on the basis of microcalcifications alone. Andersson (1980) found calcifications were the dominant abnormality in 95% (17/18) of in situ carcinomas detected on screening mammography.

Benign and Malignant Calcifications

Although early reports suggested that clustered microcalcifications associated with benign and malignant disease have certain distinguishing characteristics (Gershon-Cohen et al. 1962, 1966), later studies involving a larger number of cases indicated that considerable overlapping exists (Egan et al. 1980; Lanyi 1985). The major criteria which have been used to distinguish malignant from benign calcifications include size, shape, contour, number, distribution, and spatial relationship.

Although the initial studies of Leborgne (1949, 1951) described malignant microcalcifications as "tiny, dot-like, and resembling fine grains of salt," subsequent investigators were unable reliably to separate calcifications of less than 2 mm into benign or malignant types on the basis of their size (Millis et al. 1976; Murphy and DeSchryver-Kecskemeti

Table 1. Percentage of nonpalpable cancers detected by microcalcifications alone

Author	Percentage
Wolfe (1974)	37% (52/139)
Frischbier and Lohbeck (1977)	29% (18/62)
Feig et al. (1977)	47% (28/60)
Bjurstam (1978)	37% (10/27)
Menges et al. (1981)	48% (106/220)
Frankl and Ackerman (1983)	35% (111/321)

1978; Egan et al. 1980; Martin 1982). Although some experts (Egan et al. 1980; Tabár and Dean 1983) consider variation in size as suggestive of malignancy, this criterion is often hard to apply due to the small size of the particles and resolution limitations of the imaging system.

A thin, splinter-like microlinear shape (width ≤ 1 mm and length ≤ 3 mm) or a crystalline angulated shape is generally considered to be suspicious for ductal carcinoma (Hoeffken and Lanyi 1977; Martin 1982; Wolfe 1983). However, this appearance may also be seen in some benign ductal conditions such as papillomatosis. Round or oval shapes are nonspecific; they may be either benign or malignant.

An irregular shape, contour or margin of the calcification is suggestive of malignancy to some investigators (Sigfússon et al. 1983; Tabár and Dean 1983; Wolfe 1983) but not to others (Martin 1982; Bjurstam 1978; Millis et al. 1976). Smooth-bordered calcifications do not necessarily imply a benign process unless they are round, uniform density spheres of 2 mm or more (Moskowitz 1979; Egan et al. 1980; Sigfússon et al. 1983).

Similarly, although malignant calcifications have been described as typically dense (Hoeffken and Lanyi 1977), Millis et al. (1976) believe there is no radiologic density difference between benign and malignant particles. Variations in density among calcific particles and within individual particles seem to suggest malignancy to some investigators (Hoeffken and Lanyi 1977; Tabár and Dean 1983) but not to others (Murphy and DeSchryver-Kecskemeti 1978; Egan et al. 1980).

Several studies (Rogers and Powell 1972; Menges et al. 1973; Egan et al. 1980; Muir et al. 1983) show a correlation between the number of calcifications in a cluster and the likelihood of a malignancy. This criterion has found practical application to clusters containing less than $5-10$ microcalcifications/cm^2 where the chance of malignancy may be less than seen in lesions containing more microcalcifications. Bjurstam (1978) states that clusters of less than 5 microcalcifications/cm^2 are so common that he does not consider them as being of diagnostic significance. Sigfússon et al. (1983) usually advise follow-up rather than immediate surgical biopsy on clusters of less than five microcalcifications. However, Millis et al. (1976) did not find any such correlation. Wolfe (1983), though acknowledging that the usual case of carcinoma has at least $10-15$ deposits, does not feel that a certain number of calcifications should be necessary before biopsy is advised. His determination is more heavily based on the morphology of the deposits and their relationship to one another.

Distribution and spatial relationship are generally acknowledged to be extremely helpful guides to the need for biopsy. Malignant calcifications are usually clustered and unilateral (Hoeffken and Lanyi 1977; Martin 1982; Tabár and Dean 1983) whereas benign calcifications are usually bilateral and symmetrically distributed. A linear or branching arrangement or one which is irregular and does not conform to anatomic planes is particularly suspicious for malignancy (Hoeffken and Lanyi 1977; Moskowitz 1979; Martin 1982; Sigfússon et al. 1983).

In many cases, calcifications will appear sufficiently malignant or benign so that biopsy is definitely indicated or contraindicated. In other instances, the distinction may not be clear cut. Their appearance may suggest the possibility of carcinoma to varying degrees. A review of the literature reveals one malignancy among three cases biopsied for calcifications (Table 2). Thus, they are sensitive but not specific cancer markers. Although certain types and patterns of calcifications are pathognomonic of a benign process while others provide a highly reliable indication of malignancy, many are indeterminate.

The observation that benign and malignant calcifications may be difficult or impossible to distinguish is not surprising considering that adenosis and papillomatosis, benign

Table 2. Percentage of clustered microcalcifications which are malignant on biopsy

Author	Percentage
Bjurstam (1978)	27% (15/56)
Burphy and DeSchryver-Kecskemeti (1978)	35% (11/31)
Egan et al. (1980)	25% (115/468)
Sickles (1980)	36% (57/160)
Muir et al. (1983)	38% (17/45)
Sigfússon (1983)	33% (70/213)
Schwartz et al. (1984)	33% (104/320)

entities which provide the link between normal and cancerous tissue (Gallager and Martin 1969 a, 1969 b), frequently calcify. Another explanation must surely be that some characteristics used to distinguish benign and malignant microcalcifications may not be accurately evaluated from a routine mammogram. For example, studies with limited magnification ($1.5 \times$) show that one criterion, calcifications/cm^2, will vary according to the resolution of the recording system (Sickles 1980). Thus, with improved resolution from magnification (Sickles 1980) or grid (McSweeney et al. 1983), it may be possible to exclude more benign lesions from biopsy. It is also possible that conventional radiographic images already contain diagnostic information that may not be appreciated because the images are relatively small.

Magnification Methods

Several authors have described the use of direct radiographic magnification to obtain enlarged images (Sickles 1979, 1980). With this technique, however, magnifications exceeding $1.5 \times -2.0 \times$ are precluded because of the need for increased radiation dose to the patient and because of inherent limitations with respect to focal spot size and tube loading characteristics in state-of-the-art mammographic equipment.

Previously, we reported another technique for obtaining magnified images of breast calcifications (Frasca et al. 1981 a, 1981 b) in which the images in a small section of the radiograph are magnified with a scanning electron microscope. Although magnifications greater than $200 \times$ can be obtained with no additional radiation dose to the patient, this technique is also of limited usefulness because it requires expensive equipment and a specially trained operator, because the process is time consuming, and because only a small area of the radiograph can be examined at once.

More recently, we demonstrated that good-quality magnified images of breast calcifications can be obtained from specimen radiographs with an optical dissecting microscope (Galkin et al. 1982, 1983) (Fig. 1). If no hard copy image is needed, the specimen radiograph is positioned under the microscrope and the magnified image is directly observed. The degree of magnification is continuously adjustable up to $180 \times$.

This method has several advantages over both direct radiographic magnification and scanning electron microscopy, i.e., there is no additional radiation dose to the patient, the equipment is inexpensive, the process is quick, and magnifications up to $180 \times$ can be obtained easily by the radiologist. A permanent record of the magnified image, a photomicrograph, can be obtained by means of a camera attached to the microscope.

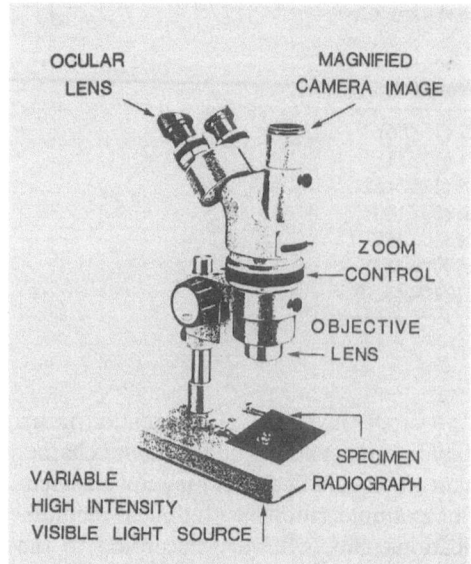

Fig. 1. Schematic for obtaining highly magnified images from radiographs. The high-intensity light source is not shown

Optical Magnification Technique

To obtain photomicrographs such as those seen in Figs. 2–15, the specimen radiograph is photographed through an optical zoom-stereo dissecting microscope onto 35-mm film and the photos are then enlarged with a darkroom enlarger. The process proceeds as follows: (1) A quick visual scan of the radiograph is made with the microscope at low magnification (7.0 ×) to locate the calcifications. (2) An area of calcifications is selected and photographed on 35-mm film at low magnification (less than 20 ×). This small degree of enlargement is used to stay below the region of "empty magnification" imposed by the microscope lenses. In both step 1 and step 2, the intensity of the light transmitted through the radiograph is a critical factor and is controlled by adjusting a special variable-intensity light source. (3) The 35-mm film is hand developed using Eastman Kodak Company's recommended chemistry. (4) Final magnification (generally 15 × –50 ×) is achieved by enlarging the 35-mm negative with a darkroom enlarger and Kodak XTL film. The resulting enlargement is developed in a 90-s automatic processor using regular chemistry.

Results

The photomicrographs reveal many features of breast calcifications that are difficult to appreciate from their unmagnified images. The borders of an individual calcification may be irregular (Fig. 2) or well defined (Fig. 3). Many distinct shapes were observed which varied from round (Fig. 3) to oval (Fig. 4), rhomboidal (Fig. 5), linear and curvilinear (Fig. 6), highly angulated Z (Fig. 7), bean-like or constricted, less well characterized amorphous (Figs. 8, 9), and crab-like or serpentine (Fig. 10) shapes.

Large-field examination frequently revealed repetitive patterns within the same specimen (Figs. 5, 6, 11). Cases where calcifications were elongated (Figs. 6, 12), highly angulated (Fig. 7), or linearly arrayed (Fig. 13) were nearly always malignant. Well-defined round or oval calcifications were usually benign (Figs. 3, 4, 11), but some malignant calcifications

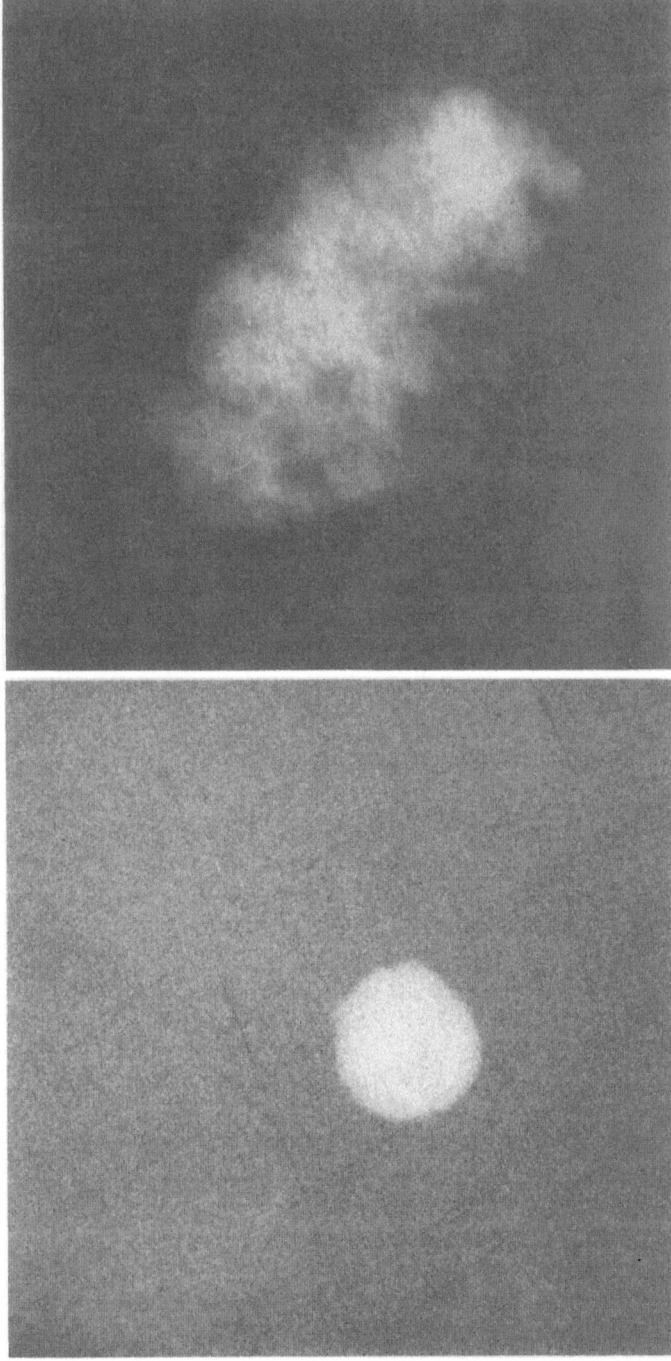

Fig. 2 *(above).* Irregular borders. Calcified papilloma, X 40

Fig. 3 *(below).* Smooth borders, round. Fibrocystic disease, X 21

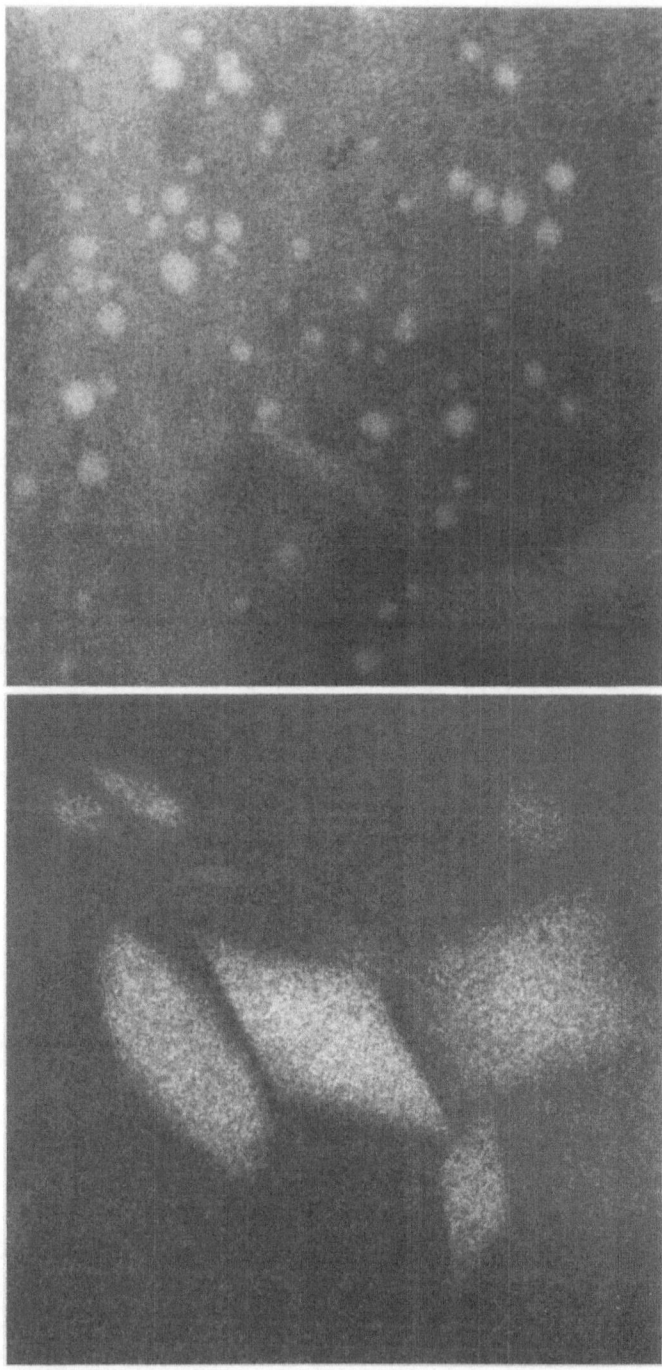

Fig. 4 *(above).* Multiple round and oval microcalcifications. Sclerosing adenosis, X 15

Fig. 5 *(below).* Rhomboidal shape. Fibrocystic disease, X 50

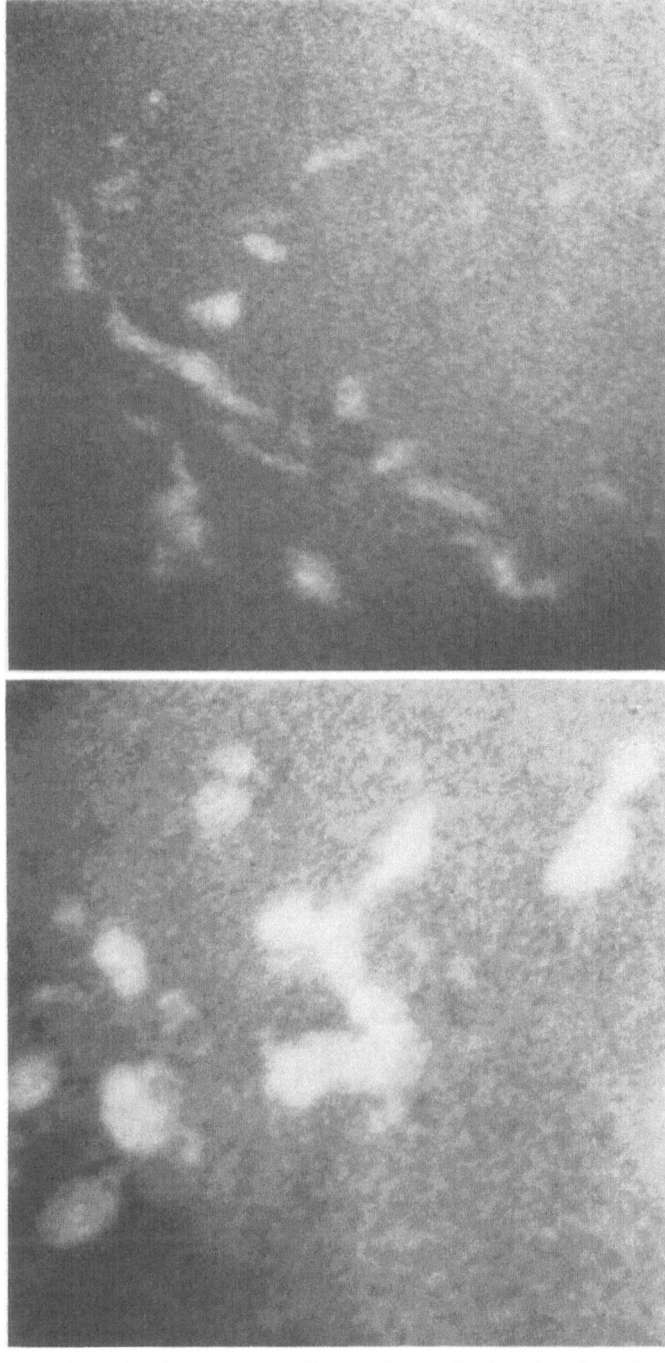

Fig. 6 *(above)*. Linear and curvilinear shapes. In situ ductal carcinoma, X 18

Fig. 7 *(below)*. Highly angulated Z shape. Infiltrating duct carcinoma, X 21

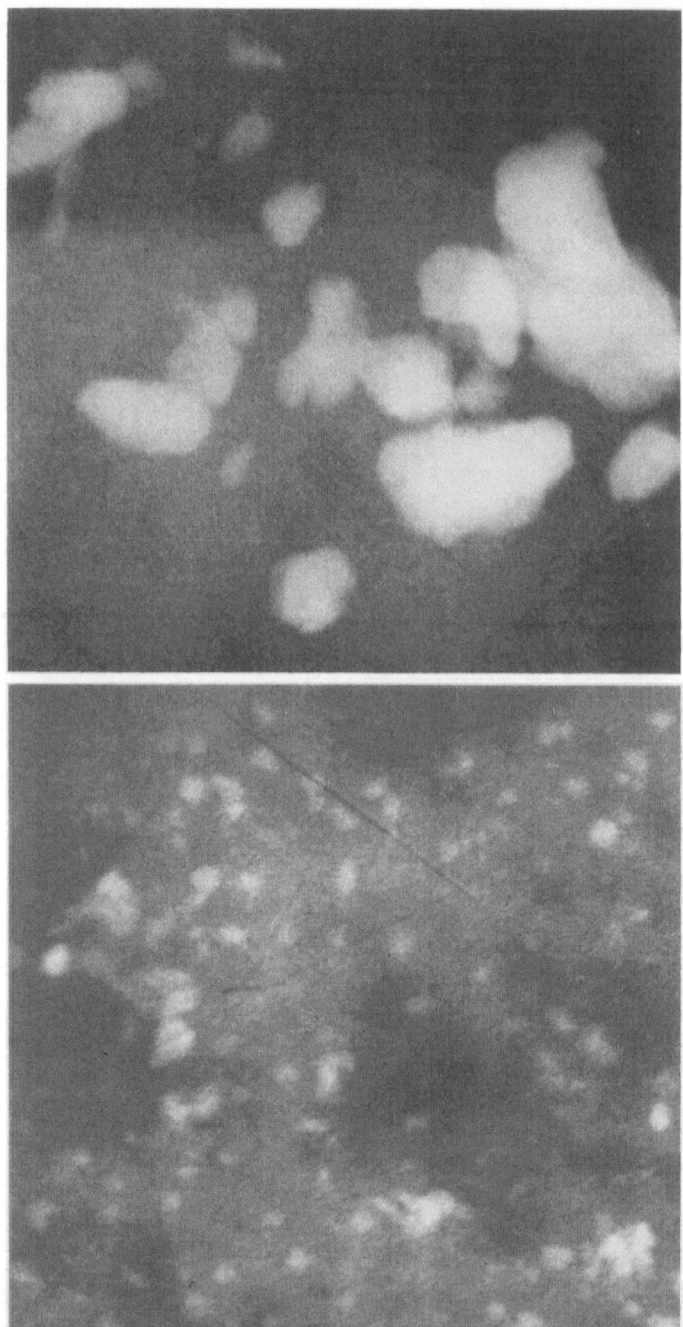

Fig. 8 *(above)*. Amorphous shapes. Fibrocystic disease with focal papillomatosis, X 15

Fig. 9 *(below)*. Amorphous shapes. Intraductal carcinoma, X 14

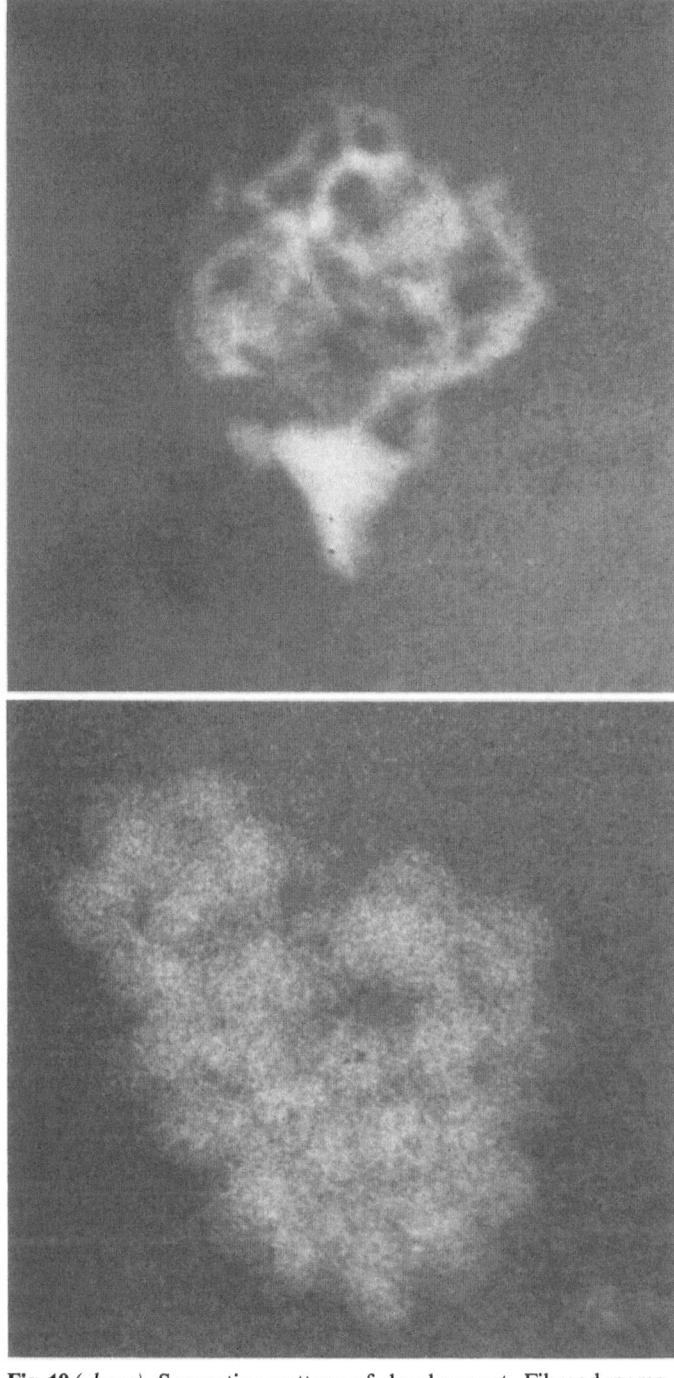

Fig. 10 *(above)*. Serpentine pattern of development. Fibroadenoma, X 21

Fig. 11 *(below)*. Tightly packed round and oval calcifications. Fibrocystic disease, X 60

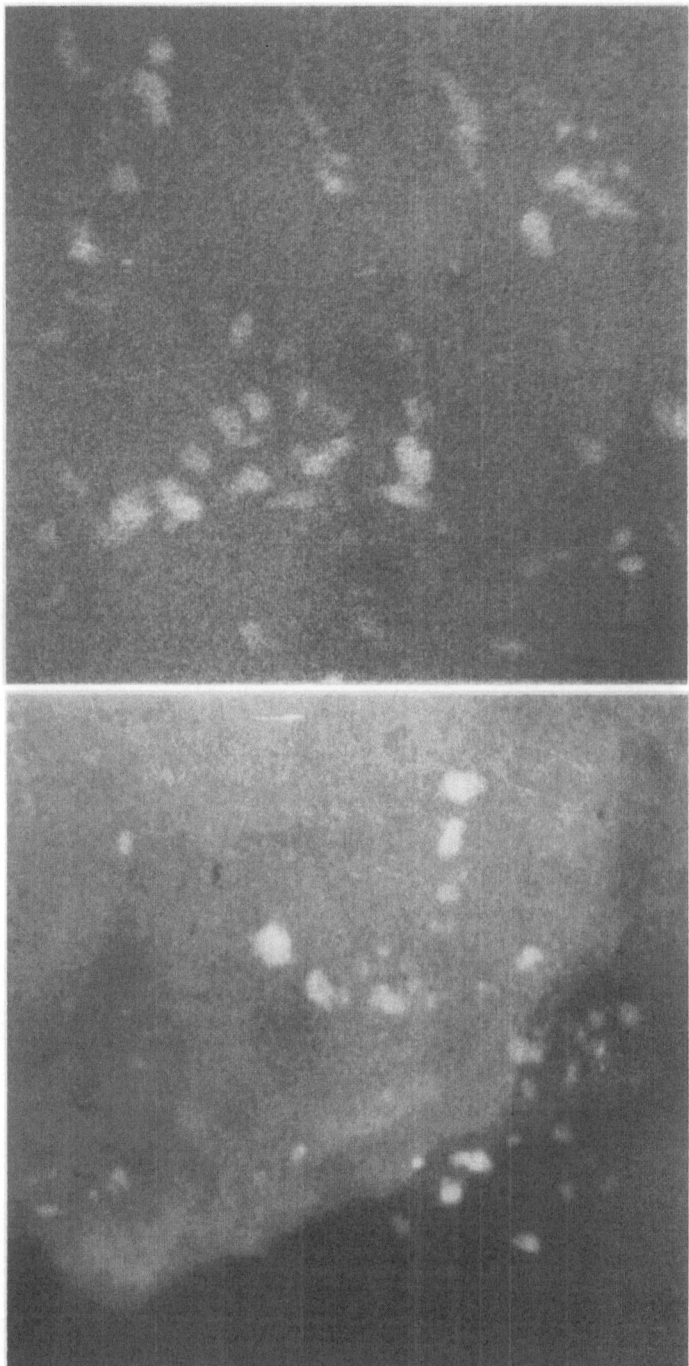

Fig. 12 *(above)*. Elongated calcifications. In situ and invasive ductal carcinoma, X 14

Fig. 13 *(below)*. Linearly arrayed calcifications. In situ and invasive duct carcinoma, X 14

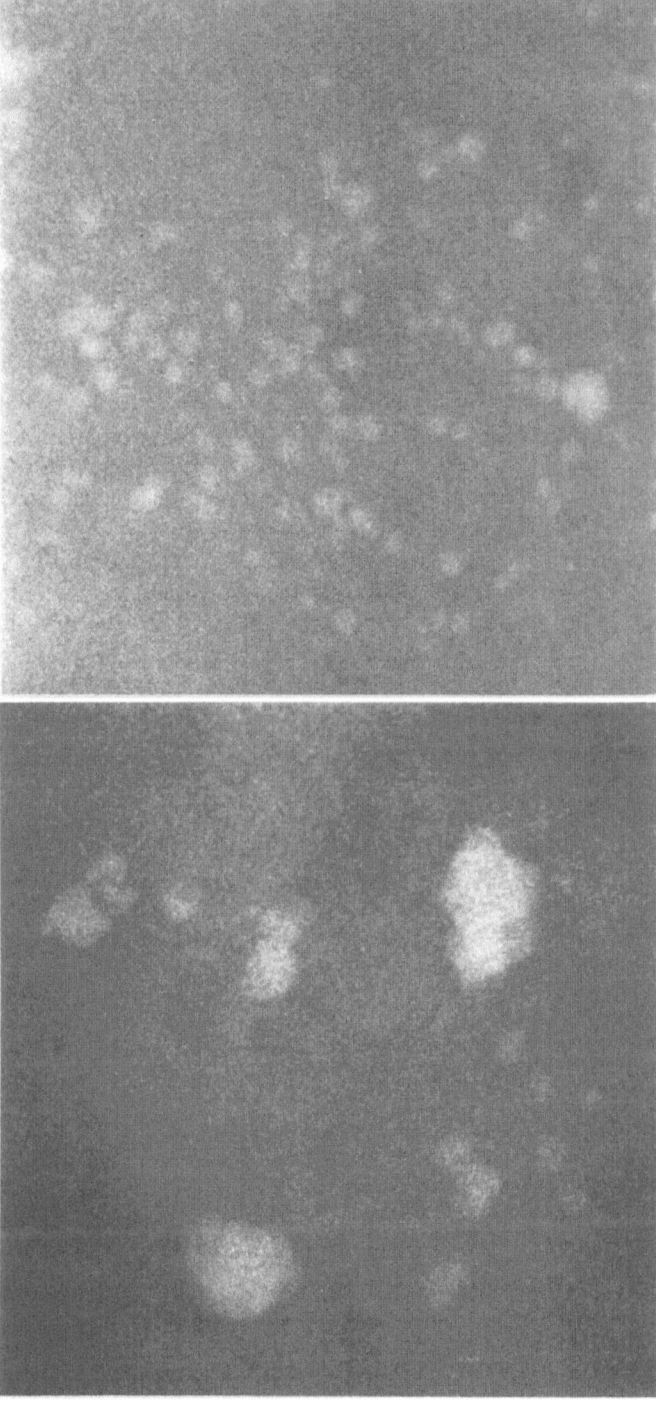

Fig. 14 *(above)*. Multiple round and oval calcifications. In situ and infiltrating duct carcinoma, X 20

Fig. 15 *(below)*. Nonspecific-appearing calcifications. Infiltrating duct carcinoma, X 14

(Fig. 14) were indistinguishable. Calcifications which generally lacked a characteristic shape were either benign (Fig. 8) or malignant (Figs. 9, 15).

Additional examples of optically enlarged images of microcalcifications were previously reported by us (Galkin et al. 1983). Subsequently, Lanyi (1985b) described four recurring forms of microcalcifications: punctiform, bean form, undulating of various lengths, and branching form or V, W, X, Y, or Z form as seen following optical projection with 20 × magnification.

Conclusion

The extent to which microscopic magnification can be applied to mammographic diagnosis, i.e., before biopsy, remains to be determined. In conventional mammograms, the images of the calcifications may not be as sharp as in specimen radiographs because of screen-film blur and penumbra. In xeromammograms (where the same magnification technique can be used, but with reflected light instead of transmitted light), loss of detail could occur because of edge enhancement and toner shape. Moreover, a particular calcification or a group of calcifications can appear with various shapes depending on the geometry of the system used in obtaining the radiographs.

Nevertheless, the photomicrographs show that additional diagnostic information about breast calcifications is contained in the radiographs. Such information might augment or replace present diagnostic criteria and improve diagnostic accuracy.

We are currently involved in a multi-institutional study to determine if the additional information contained in optically magnified specimen radiographs can increase the specificity of mammographic diagnosis. If differences between benign and malignant calcifications cannot be found on optical magnification, then it stands to reason that such differences cannot be perceived on the routine nonmagnified image. On the other hand, if criteria for diagnosing benign from malignant calcifications can be appreciated on optical magnification, then such criteria might be tested for possible application to current or improved mammographic techniques.

References

Andersson I (1980) Mammographic screening for breast carcinoma. (Thesis) Sigillum Universitatis Gothor Caroline Lund. Malmö, Sweden
Bjurstam N (1978) Radiology of the female breast and axilla. Acta Radiol Suppl No. 357
Egan RL, McSweeney MB, Sewell CW (1980) Intramammary calcifications without an associated mass in benign and malignant diseases. Radiology 137: 1-7
Feig SA, Shaber GS, Patchefsky A, et al (1977) Analysis of clinically occult and mammographically occult breast tumors. AJR 128: 403-408
Frankl G, Ackerman M (1983) Xeromammography and 1200 breast cancers. Radiol Clin North Am 21: 81-91
Frasca P, Galkin BM, Feig SA (1981a) A new no-dose method to improve mammographic detail using scanning electron microscopy - a possible aid in the diagnosis of breast cancer (Abst.). Medical Physics 8: 563
Frasca P, Galkin BM, Feig SA, et al (1981b) A new method of magnifying photographic image using the scanning electron microscope in the backscattered electron detection mode. In: Johari O (ed) Scanning electron microscopy. SEM Inc., AMF O'Hare, Chicago, pp 917-923
Frischbier H-J, Lohbeck HU (1977) Frühdiagnostik des Mammakarzinoms. Thieme, Stuttgart
Galkin BM, Frasca P, Feig SA, et al (1982) Magnified radiographic images using optical compound microscopes (Abst.). Med Phys 9: 648

Galkin BM, Feig SA, Frasca P, et al (1983) Photomicrographs of breast calcifications: correlation with histopathologic diagnosis. RadioGraphics 3: 450–477

Gallager HS, Martin JE (1969 a) The study of mammary carcinoma by mammography and whole organ sectioning. Early observations. Cancer 23: 855–873

Gallager HS, Martin JE (1969 b) Early phases in the development of breast cancer. Cancer 24: 1170–1178

Gershon-Cohen J, Yiu LS, Berger SM (1962) The diagnostic importance of calcareous patterns in roentgenography of breast cancer. AJR 88: 1117–1125

Gershon-Cohen J, Berger SM, Curcio BM (1966) Breast cancer with microcalcifications: diagnostic difficulties. Radiology 87: 613–622

Hoeffken W, Lanyi M (1977) Mammography. Saunders, Philadelphia

Lanyi M (1985 a) Microcalcifications in the breast – a blessing or a curse? Diagn Imag Clin Med 54: 126–145

Lanyi M (1985 b) Morphologic analysis of microcalcifications. In: Zander J, Baltzer J (eds) Early breast cancer. Springer, Berlin Heidelberg New York Tokyo, pp 113–135

Leborgne R, Dominguez CM, Mautone JA (1949) Diagnóstico de los tumores de la mama por la radiografía simple. Boletin de la Sociedad de Cirugia del Uruguay 20: 407–422

Leborgne R (1951) Diagnosis of tumors of the breast by simple roentgenography: calcifications in carcinomas. AJR 65: 1–11

Martin J (1982) Atlas of mammography. Williams and Wilkins, Baltimore

McSweeney MB, Sprawls P, Egan RL (1983) Mammographic grids. In: Feig SA, McLelland R (eds) Breast carcinoma: current diagnosis and treatment. Masson, New York, pp 169–176

Menges V, Wellauer J, Engeler V, et al (1973) Korrelation zahlenmäßig erfaßter Mikroverkalkungen auf dem Mammogram und dadurch diagnostizierter Carcinome und Mastopathietypen. Radologe 13: 468–476

Menges V, Busing CM, Hirsch O (1981) Die diagnostische Wertigkeit einer einzelnen Malignitatszeichen des klinisch okkulten Mammakarzinoms in Mammogram. RoFo 135: 372–378

Millis RR, Davis R, Stacey AJ (1976) The detection and significance of calcifications in the breast: a radiological and pathological study. Br J Radiol 49: 12–26

Moskowitz M (1979) Screening is not diagnosis. Radiology 133: 265–268

Moskowitz M (1983) The predictive value of certain mammographic signs in screening for breast cancer. Cancer 51: 1007–1011

Muir BB, Lamb J, Anderson TJ, et al (1983) Microcalcification and its relationship to cancer of the breast: experience in a screening clinic. Clin Radiol 34: 193–200

Murphy WA, DeSchryver-Kecskemeti K (1978) Isolated clustered microcalcifications in the breast: radiologic-pathologic correlation. Radiology 127: 335–341

Rogers JV, Powell RW (1972) Mammographic indications for biopsy of clinically normal breasts. Correlation with pathologic findings in 72 cases. AJR 115: 794–800

Salomon A (1913) Beiträge zur Pathologie und Klinik der Mammakarzinome. Arch Klin Chir 101: 573–668

Schwartz GF, Feig SA, Rosenberg AL, et al (1984) Staging and treatment of clinically occult breast cancer. Cancer 53: 1379–1384

Sickles EA (1979) Microfocal spot magnification mammography using xeroradiographic and screen-film recording systems. Radiology 131: 599–607

Sickles EA (1980) Further experience with microfocal spot magnification mammography in assessment of clustered breast microcalcifications. Radiology 137: 9–14

Sigfússon BF, Andersson I, Aspegren K, et al (1983) Clustered breast calcifications. Acta Radiologica 24: 273–281

Tabár L, Dean PB (1983) Teaching atlas of mammography. Thieme, Stuttgart

Wolfe JN (1974) Analysis of 462 breast carcinomas. AJR 121: 846–853

Wolfe JN (1983) Xeroradiography of the breast. Thomas, Springfield

Contributions to the Diagnosis of Contralateral Malignancies in Women with Invasive Breast Cancer

M. Nielsen, L. Christensen, U. Dyreborg, and J. A. Andersen

Department of Pathology, Frederiksberg Hospital, 2000 F Copenhagen, Denmark

Introduction

Women with breast cancer are at a high risk of developing a new primary or metastatic lesion in the contralateral breast (Robbins and Berg 1964; Haagensen 1971; Leis 1980). The magnitude of this risk and the prognostic significance of the occurrence of such lesions, however, remain controversial. Discriminants of predictive value for the development of contralateral malignancies are a matter of debate as well and there is no general agreement on the management of the contralateral breast (Leis 1980; Fisher et al. 1984).

The increasing detection of contralateral malignancies, simultaneous or subsequent, is undoubtedly due to the increased use of mammography and simultaneous breast biopsies (Egan 1976; Gutter 1976; Urban et al. 1977). It is generally accepted that in the absence of palpable and/or gross lesions the result of the pathologic examination of the breast may be improved considerably by specimen radiography as a guide to tissue sampling for microscopy (Rosen 1980; Snyder 1980; Holland 1985).

In a recent autopsy study of 84 women with invasive breast cancer the overall frequency of malignancies of the contralateral breast was as high as 80% (Nielsen et al. 1986). Fifty-seven women (68%) had a new primary cancer and 13 women (16%) had metastatic tumors, 12 from the earlier ipsilateral breast cancer. On the basis of this material the value of various diagnostic procedures for detection of contralateral malignancies is presented.

Material

Our study included 84 consecutive, unselected autopsy cases of women with known invasive breast cancer from Frederiksberg Hospital and Glostrup County Hospital, both in the Copenhagen area. The autopsies were performed from 1982 to 1984. During this period almost 65% of the total number of deaths within the metropolitan area occurred during hospital admission and the autopsy rate in the two hospitals was 75% and 50%, respectively.

The age distribution and clinical staging of the first cancer did not differ from Danish national figures.

The treatment of the ipsilateral cancer was in accordance with common practice in Denmark. Ninety-two percent of the women had had mastectomy. Eighty percent had received local radiotherapy, and treatment with cytotoxic chemotherapy and/or tamoxifen had been carried out in 56% of the cases.

Patient selection may result from the method of referral, the type of hospital, and other variables which may be expected to contribute to the variation in the reported frequencies

Recent Results in Cancer Research. Vol 105
© Springer-Verlag Berlin · Heidelberg 1987

of contralateral malignancy. As the cases in our study were consecutive and unselected the material may be assumed to be a representative sample of Danish women dying in general hospitals following a diagnosis of invasive breast cancer.

The main histologic findings are summarized in Table 1.

Table 1. Histologic features of primary invasive and in situ breast cancer of the contralateral breast

Type of carcinoma	No. of women	Microfocal	Tumor forming[a]	Multicentric[b]
Invasive ductal	20	5	15	14
Invasive lobular	7	1	6	5
Invasive mucinous	1	–	1	1
DCIS	17	17	–	7
LCIS	3	3	–	2
DCIS and LCIS	9	9	–	8[c]
Total	57	35	22	37

DCIS, intraductal carcinoma; *LCIS*, lobular carcinoma in situ.
[a] Tumor forming: the diameter of the lesion exceeded 5 mm.
[b] Multicentricity: separate foci of lesions in more than one quadrant.
[c] Three of these lesions were diffuse, i.e., multiple microfocal lesions in one or more quadrants.

Clinical Examination

Frequently, as in the present study, no systematic follow-up program is established for the contralateral breast at the regular clinical examinations after initial treatment of the ipsilateral cancer. As with the first cancer, early diagnosis must be expected to ensure a good prognosis. Experience shows, however, that contralateral cancers are often detected incidentially by the woman herself or at a routine clinical checkup and not at a particularly early stage (Robbins and Berg 1964; Leis 1980).

In our study only 10 women were suspected clinically of having contralateral malignancy. Two of them had mastectomy performed for a new invasive primary, clinical stage I and II, respectively. None of the eight other women had received any surgical treatment as a consequence of the clinical finding because of advanced clinical stage. At the postmortem examination five of these untreated women had invasive primaries, three with involvement of the axillary lymph nodes, one had in situ cancer of diffuse ductal type, and another had both microfocal ductal in situ cancer and a breast metastasis. One woman had no contralateral malignancy.

The frequency of clinically detected cancers in the present study corresponds well with the findings of others (Robbins and Berg 1964; Urban et al. 1977; Fisher et al. 1984). However, the number comprised only 25% of all the invasive contralateral primaries discovered histologically at autopsy. For the 67 women in the series with histologically proven malignant changes this means that the majority (87%) had clinically occult lesions.

Nine women had palpable axillary lymph nodes on the contralateral side. In three cases the lymph node involvement was thought clinically to be spread from the second tumor, but histologic examination revealed it to be metastases from the contralateral primaries in the majority of the nine cases.

Radiologic Examination

As a result of improved techniques for clinical mammography it has been advocated with increasing frequency that women with breast cancer should have the contralateral breast examined periodically not only by physical but also by mammographic methods (McSweeney and Egan 1984). Mammography has proved valuable not only in the diagnosis of an increasing number of malignancies but also in the detection of the lesions at a more favorable clinical stage (Beahrs and Smart 1979).

At the hospitals participating in the present study, clinical mammography was used only as a specific diagnostic procedure and not as a screening examination. Only four of the women had had a clinical mammography of the contralateral breast. Two of these women had a new primary diagnosed and treated. The other two had changes interpreted as fibrocystic disease, but at the postmortem examination 22 and 25 months later an in situ and an invasive primary cancer were found, respectively, both now with typical radiologic and histologic appearances.

Each intact breast specimen from the 71 autopsies from Frederiksberg Hospital was radiographied in a single, frontal projection. The examination was performed immediately after removal in a Faxitron (model 43805N) using Kodak industrial M film. The model has a fixed target-to-film distance and constant milliamperage of 3 mA, whereas its kilovoltage and exposure time may be varied. The X-ray films were later evaluated blindly by one of the authors (U. D.).

The radiologic findings at the postmortem examination are shown in Table 2. Of the 24 women with in situ cancer, 11 (46%) had clusters of microcalcifications and six (25%) had soft tissue density with or without microcalcifications. Of the 22 women with invasive primaries 15 (70%) had soft tissue densities and two (9%) had only clustered microcalcifications. These radiologic changes would during a life time have called for a breast biopsy in 71% and 77% of the women with in situ and invasive primaries, respectively. Half of the 12 women with breast metastases had soft tissue densities without calcifications. Thus, among the 58 women with malignant changes examined by specimen radiography and clinical mammography, 42 (72%) had changes suggestive of breast malignancy in the areas

Table 2. Radiologic findings on the contralateral breast in 69 women at the postmortem examination

	In situ carcinoma		Invasive carcinoma		Breast metastasis	No malignant changes
Microcalcifications	11	7 DCIS, 4 DCIS and LCIS	2	1 mucinous, T, 1 lobular, T	–	3
Soft tissue density +/− calcifications	6	3 DCIS, 3 DCIS and LCIS	15	10 ductal, T 1 ductal, M 4 lobular, T	6	2
No radiologic changes	7	1 LCIS, 6 DCIS	5	2 lobular, T 1 ductal, T 2 ductal, M	6	8
No. of women[a]	24		22		12	13

DCIS, intraductal carcinoma; *LCIS*, lobular carcinoma in situ; *T*, tumor with a diameter exceeding 5 mm; *M*, tumor with a diameter less than 5 mm.
[a] Two women had both breast metastasis and in situ carcinoma.

with histologically proven malignancies. Of the 49 women with clinically occult lesions specimen radiography raised suspicion of a contralateral malignancy in as many as 58%. This frequency, however, cannot be directly compared with the favorable results of other investigations using specimen radiography due to the character of our study. Among the 18 false-negative cases seven were microfocal in situ cancers with no mass component or calcifications and thus impossible to detect on the mammogram.

Pathologic Examination

For the pathologic examination a contralateral total mastectomy with partial axillary dissection *ad modum* Cady (1973) was performed in all cases except for the two women who had had bilateral mastectomy. All glandular tissue and all lymph nodes were systematically examined and serially sliced, and after fixation in formalin all the tissue was processed for paraffin embedding. Sections for histologic evaluation were cut and stained with hematoxylin and eosin from a total of 19 265 paraffin blocks, varying from 39 to 1245 per breast specimen.

At the gross examination malignant changes were suspected in only 13 breast specimens. Furthermore, lymph node metastases were suspected in five cases of the 31 women with positive contralateral axillary lymph nodes. The remaining histologically proven malignant cases (68%) were not detected by gross inspection and palpation.

Table 1 lists the types and different growth patterns of the primary cancers. Twenty-eight women (33%) had primary invasive cancer and another 29 women (35%) had in situ lesions.

A contralateral invasive primary was diagnosed if the tumor was of another histologic type than the ipsilateral or if the tumor was intimately associated with in situ lesions. All other invasive cancers were considered metastatic spread.

Metastases to the regional axillary lymph nodes and distant metastases occurred significantly more frequently in women with invasive contralateral primaries than in women with in situ cancer or no malignant changes (Table 3).

Thus, our study demonstrated a very high frequency of the lifelong cumulated contralateral malignancies compared with most other investigations (Robbins and Berg 1964; Haagensen 1971; Leis 1980). About one-third of the lesions were only found by the histologic examination, whereas clinical evaluation and/or radiologic examination showed indicative changes in the remaining cases. The few other studies with comparable high frequencies of contralateral malignancies have been based on the use of random biopsies (Urban et al. 1977) or extensive histopathologic examination (Ringberg et al. 1982; Alpers and Wellings 1985).

Table 3. Regional axillary lymph node metastases and distant metastases in women with contralateral breast carcinoma

	No. of women	Node metastases	Distant metastases
New contralateral invasive carcinoma	28	20 (71%) $\rangle P < 0.002$	22 (79%) $\rangle P < 0.001$
None	56	11 (20%)	23 (41%)

Table 4. Death of disseminated breast cancer in relation to a new contralateral invasive breast cancer

	No. of women	Death of disseminated breast cancer
New contralateral invasive cancer	28	21 (75%)
None	56	17 (30%)

$P < 0.001$

Survival

There have been conflicting opinions concerning the prognostic significance of the occurrence of a contralateral malignancy (Robbins and Berg 1964; Leis 1980; Fisher et al. 1984). Many authors, however, find that a second breast cancer is an additional risk to the woman and should be detected at a stage at which treatment might still eliminate their threat (Leis 1980).

The median survival for all the women in the present series was 9 years after diagnosis of the ipsilateral cancer. Surprisingly, the life expectancy of women with and without new invasive primaries was similar (5-year survival of 50% and 52%, respectively). Women with an invasive contralateral primary, however, had a significantly higher risk of dying from disseminated disease than women without such lesions (Table 4). Similarly, breast cancer continued to be a cause of death in the group of women with invasive contralateral cancer for the rest of their lives whereas this ceased after 11 years in women with in situ or no cancer of the contralateral breast.

Predictive Factors

None of the predictive factors proposed in the literature (Robbins and Berg 1964; Haagensen 1971; Leis 1980; Fisher et al. 1984) such as histologic type, size, clinical staging, degree of anaplasia, and location of the ipsilateral cancer were found to be of value regarding the cumulated risk of developing contralateral breast cancer. No influence of a family history of breast cancer, age, parity, estrogen therapy or treatment with cytotoxic drugs or tamoxifen could be demonstrated either. The lifetime risk of contralateral breast cancer was also independent of the length of survival. The risk per year, however, tended to be decreased in long-term survivors.

The significance of ipsilateral radiotherapy for development of contralateral malignancy could not be evaluated as most of the women had had this treatment.

Fibrocystic disease (including parameters such as radial scar and papilloma) of the contralateral breast was the only factor registered to be significantly associated with contralateral primaries, invasive as well as in situ cancers. Fibrocystic disease occurred in 70% of the breasts with contralateral cancer and in only 19% of breasts without. Because of the known bilateral occurrence of fibrocystic disease, ipsilateral fibrocystic disease might also be expected to be a predictive factor (Kiær 1954). This possibility, however, could not be evaluated because too little breast tissue was available in a large proportion of the cases. For the same reasons the importance of multicentricity of the ipsilateral breast tumor could not be evaluated. However, an association with contralateral primaries was suggested from the material present (20% were multicentric and of these 96% were associated with a new contralateral cancer).

Conclusions

1. The lifelong cumulated frequency of malignancies in the contralateral breast is high in women with clinical invasive breast cancer.
2. The biologic significance of contralateral breast cancer is indicated by the fact that second invasive primaries are significantly correlated to regional axillary lymph node metastases and death from disseminated breast cancer.
3. Fibrocystic disease and multicentric breast cancer may be predictive factors for the development of primary malignancy on the contralateral side.
4. Specimen radiography is a valuable tool in detecting clinically occult contralateral malignancies of the breast.
5. The many clinically occult contralateral malignancies suggest that systematic physical examinations and repeated mammography of the second breast following diagnosis of the first breast cancer may improve the diagnosis.

References

Alpers CE, Wellings SE (1985) The prevalence of carcinoma in situ in normal and cancer-associated breasts. Hum Path 16: 796–807
Beahrs OH, Smart CR (1979) Diagnosis of minimal breast cancers in the BCDDP. Cancer 43: 848–850
Cady B (1973) Total mastectomy and partial axillary dissection. Surg Clin North Am 53: 313–318
Egan RL (1976) Bilateral breast carcinomas. Role of mammography. Cancer 38: 931–938
Fisher ER, Fisher B, Sass R, Wickerham L, Collaborating NSABP Investigators (1984) Pathologic findings from the national surgical adjuvant breast project (Protocol No. 4). Cancer 54: 3002–3011
Gutter Z (1976) Cancer of the remaining breast: radiologic contribution to diagnosis. Can Med Assoc J 114: 27–30
Haagensen CD (1971) Diseases of the breast, 2nd edn. Saunders, Philadelphia, pp 449–458
Holland R, Veling SHJ, Mravunac M, Hendriks JHCL (1985) Histologic multifocality of Tis, T1-2 breast carcinomas. Cancer 56: 979–990
Kiær W (1954) Relation of fibroadenomatosis ("chronic mastitis") to cancer of the breast. Munksgaard, Copenhagen
Leis HP (1980) Managing the remaining breast. Cancer 46: 1026–1030
McSweeney MB, Egan RL (1985) Bilateral breast carcinoma. In: Brünner S, Langfeldt B, Andersen PE (eds) Early detection of breast cancer. Springer, Berlin Heidelberg New York Tokyo (Recent results in cancer research, vol 90)
Nielsen M, Christensen, Andersen J (1986) Contralateral cancerous breast lesions in women with clinical invasive breast carcinoma. Cancer 57: 897–903
Ringberg A, Palmer B, Linell F (1982) The contralateral breast at reconstructive surgery after breast cancer operation: a histopathological study. Breast Cancer Res Treat 2: 151–161
Robbins GF, Berg JW (1964) Bilateral primary breast cancers. Cancer 17: 1501–1527
Rosen PP (1980) Specimen radiography and the diagnosis of clinically occult mammary carcinoma. Pathol Annu (Part I) 15: 225–236
Snyder RE (1980) Specimen radiography and preoperative localization of nonpalpable breast cancer. Cancer 46: 950–956
Urban JA, Papachristou D, Taylor J (1977) Bilateral breast cancer. Cancer 40: 1968–1973

Subject Index

A-bomb survivors 85
absorbed dose 1, 10
absorption spectra 34
air gaps 20
American cancer society-national cancer
    institute (ACS-NCI) 78
- college of radiology (ACR) 80
- medical association 80
anti-scatter grid 5
attempted excisional biopsies 103
attendance rate 62
attitudes toward mammography 73
autopsy study 124
average glandular dose 81
axillary lymph nodes 125

beam quality 48
breast biopsy 97
- cancer control 108
- - detection demonstration project
    (BCDDP) 78
- compression 15
- contrast agents 89
- pattern 107
- screening 67
- self-examination 59, 75, 80, 81

calcifications 89
"calendars" 107
chemical composition 89
chest fluoroscopy 85
clinically occult lesions 125
closed biopsy 97
coils 34
collimation 18
compliance 82
- screening guidelines 81
compression 16, 37
computed tomographic (CT) scanning 31
consensus conference 73
contralateral malignancy 124
contrast 5, 20, 53, 54
core-cutting needle 97

- - biopsy 98
costs 81

damaging effect of incisional breast biopsy 98
dedicated mammography units 15, 25
definitive diagnosis 98
density control setting 17
diagnostic quality 25
dose response models: linear, linear-quadratic,
    quadratic 86
double-coated film 45

early breast cancer 89
elements in some calcifications 89
examination costs 83
excisional biopsy 97, 103
exposure and beam quality 25
- time 16, 17

features of breast calcifications 114
fibrocystic disease 128
film contrast 40
- processing 40
- speed 16
film-screen mammography 1
fine-needle aspiration biopsy 98
Finnish cancer registry 108
focal spot 17, 19
- - size 16
- - - and shape 25
- spot-film distance (FFD) 17
frozen sections 98

geometric blurring 42
- configuration 43
grid 16, 18, 37, 40
- for mammography 39
guidelines 80
Guildford project 67

hazard of incisional biopsy 103
health insurers 83
- service costs 60